PRACTISING
CLINICAL
SUPERVISION

A REFLECTIVE APPROACH FOR HEALTHCARE PROFESSIONALS

For Elsevier:

Commissioning Editor:	Steven Black
Development Editor:	Catherine Jackson
Project Manager:	Emma Riley
Design Direction:	Sarah Russell
Illustrations:	Robert Britton, with cartoons by David Banks
Illustrations Buyer:	Merlyn Harvey

SECOND EDITION

PRACTISING CLINICAL SUPERVISION

A REFLECTIVE APPROACH FOR HEALTHCARE PROFESSIONALS

John Driscoll

BSc(Hons) DPSN CertEd(FE) RGN RMN

Professional Development Consultant & Coach
(www.supervisionandcoaching.com)

Foreword by

Tania Yegdich

Statewide Mental Health Nursing Education Advisor
Queensland Centre for Mental Health Learning (QCMHL)
Brisbane, Australia

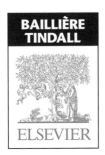

EDINBURGH LONDON NEW YORK OXFORD PHILADELPHIA ST LOUIS SYDNEY TORONTO 2007

This book is dedicated to Anne, Carly and Hayley for their continual love, support and understanding

BAILLIÈRE
TINDALL
ELSEVIER

First edition 2000
Second edition 2007

ISBN-13: 978 0 7020 2779 6
ISBN-10: 0 7020 2779 0

British Library Cataloguing in Publication Data
A catalogue record for this book is available from the British Library.

Library of Congress Cataloging in Publication Data
A catalog record for this book is available from the Library of Congress.

Note
Knowledge and best practice in this field are constantly changing. As new research and experience broaden our knowledge, changes in practice, treatment and drug therapy may become necessary or appropriate. Readers are advised to check the most current information provided (i) on procedures featured or (ii) by the manufacturer of each product to be administered, to verify the recommended dose or formula, the method and duration of administration, and contraindications. It is the responsibility of the practitioner, relying on their own experience and knowledge of the patient, to make diagnoses, to determine dosages and the best treatment for each individual patient, and to take all appropriate safety precautions. To the fullest extent of the law, neither the Publisher nor the Editor assumes any liability for any injury and/or damage to persons or property arising out or related to any use of the material contained in this book.

The Publisher

Working together to grow
libraries in developing countries

www.elsevier.com | www.bookaid.org | www.sabre.org

ELSEVIER   BOOK AID
             International   Sabre Foundation

ELSEVIER your source for books,
journals and multimedia
in the health sciences
www.elsevierhealth.com

The
Publisher's
policy is to use
**paper manufactured
from sustainable forests**

Printed in China

Contents

Section 1 – THE CONTEXT OF CLINICAL SUPERVISION

1: The place of clinical supervision in modern healthcare   3

John Driscoll & Julia O'Sullivan

Introduction; Supervisory structures in healthcare practice; The emergence of clinical supervision in healthcare settings; The purpose and functions of clinical supervision; What are your expectations for engaging in clinical supervision?; Conclusion

2: Supported reflective learning: the essence of clinical supervision?   27

John Driscoll

Introduction; Why the need to be reflective when I routinely think about what I do in my clinical practice?; How does the process of reflection relate to learning in and for practice?; How might engaging in reflection specifically support the work of the health professional?; What are some of the conditions and consequences of becoming a reflective learner in practice?; How might I incorporate some of the ideas of reflective practice into a clinical supervision situation?; Pulling it altogether: is supported reflective learning the essence of clinical supervision?

Section 2 – GETTING GOING WITH CLINICAL SUPERVISION IN PRACTICE

3: Boundaries and responsibilities in clinical supervision   53

Stephen Power

Introduction; The boundaries of clinical supervision; The clinical supervision contract

4: Essential elements for a successful supervisory partnership to flourish   72

Daniel Nicholls

Introduction; Active awareness; Choice; Communication as collaboration; Difference and similarity; Proximity — getting close — but not too close; A partnership of reflection; An interim conclusion: letting our questions stand?

Section 3 – SUPERVISORY METHODS AND APPROACHES

Section 4 – THE CONTINUING CHALLENGE OF CLINICAL SUPERVISION

Notes on the contributors

John Driscoll (Professional Development Consultant & Coach) BSc (Hons), DPSN, Cert Ed(FE), RGN, RMN
John has had extensive experience in developing clinical supervision in healthcare for over a decade in the UK and Australia. He works as a freelance professional development consultant and coach and has recently produced www.supervisionandcoaching.com as a resource website. He is particularly interested in developing appreciative and strengths-based approaches to support the organizational implementation of clinical supervision, as well as exploring alternatives to more traditional face to face encounters. Formerly a Visiting Lecturer in the School of Integrated Health at the University of Westminster in London, John now works as a part time lecturer at City College Norwich (an Associate College of the University of East Anglia). In addition, John is Continuing Professional Education (CPE) Editor for the *Journal of Orthopaedic Nursing* and joint sponsor of an annual New Writers Award for the journal in partnership with Elsevier Science.

Jeanette Hewitt (Lecturer, Centre for Mental Health Studies, University of Wales) RMN, RGN, RNT, BSc (Hons), PGCE, PG Cert Couns, Doctoral student
Jeanette has been a Lecturer in mental health nursing at the University of Wales Swansea, for the past five years. She has worked in both acute mental health settings and general adult critical care. Her research interests are in suicide, cognitive-behavioural therapy and developing therapeutic relationships. Jeanette has been involved in the development of clinical supervision for pre-registration nursing programmes and facilitates reflective groups for mental health nurses.

Berwyn Llewellyn-Davies (Clinical Supervision Project Co-ordinator Gwent Healthcare NHS Trust) RMN, Dip Community Health Studies, FETC, MA (Philosophy and Healthcare)
Berwyn became involved in clinical supervision in the 1970s when engaged in a long apprenticeship with the 'conversational model' of psychotherapy. He is currently the Trust lead for clinical supervision and has been involved in preparing staff for practice, training supervisors and developing a structure to support supervisors and maintaining clinical supervision standards. His overall aim is to embed clinical supervision as a supportive mechanism into the working culture of his organization.

Daniel Nicholls (Senior Nurse Mental Health Services Austin Health, Victoria)
RGN, RPN, PhD (Philosophy)
Daniel has been active in the development of formal clinical supervision practices for 20 years. He has introduced clinical supervision in a number of speciality and service-wide settings. In 2003 Daniel collaborated with colleagues in Victoria, Australia in the establishment of a clinical supervision conference for nurses. A second conference was held in 2005; the third is planned for April 2007. These conferences, in conjunction with educational workshops, have helped to establish a greater dialogue in Victoria around clinical supervision, which in turn has contributed to the development of state and local guidelines. Daniel favours an interdisciplinary, peer approach to clinical supervision with an emphasis on individual responsibility to engage with the process. Ultimately, he sees each clinician as having the potential, through the aid of regular reflection, for being his or her own supervisor in practice.

Daniel holds a PhD in Philosophy from Macquarie University, Sydney. He is currently the Senior Nurse of mental health services at Austin Health, Victoria.

Gerard O'Donovan (Managing Director, Noble Manhattan Coaching Ltd)
MSc, FCLC, NEBSS
Gerard is the Founder and Managing Director of Noble Manhattan Coaching Ltd, one of the largest coaching companies in Europe, whose motto is *Fortune Favours the Prepared Mind*. He is a renowned public speaker and co-author of *The Thirty Minute Life Coach* offering insights into the world of life coaching in the UK. As a strong supporter of the regulation and accreditation of coaches, Gerard actively endorses supervision as a method for ensuring the continued quality of professional coaching and as a source of ongoing support.

Julia O'Sullivan (Head of Continuing Professional Development, Chartered Society of Physiotherapy, UK) BA (Hons), MSc
Julia is responsible for developing policy and strategic direction on Continuing Professional Development (CPD) in the UK. She promotes CPD to qualified and student physiotherapists and physiotherapy support workers as well as outside bodies. A key function of her work is to provide support to enable members to undertake effective and systematic CPD through the use of guidance materials, workshops and individual advice. Julia has worked extensively with members to equip them with the skills and knowledge required for CPD, encouraging the adoption of portfolio-keeping, reflective practice and clinical supervision. Julia has undertaken research to develop strategies to support physiotherapists' CPD. She is a member of the steering group of the Inter-professional CPD Forum and has been involved in a number of government funded inter-professional CPD projects.

Stephen Power MA, BSc (Hons), PG Dip. (Ed), Dip. Psychotherapy, doctoral student
Stephen has an extensive background in psychiatric nursing, nurse education and psychodynamic psychotherapy. Having held several senior clinical and educational posts in the UK, over a twenty-five year period, he now lives in County Limerick, Ireland. He is a senior lecturer with the National Counselling Institute of Ireland (NCII) and works in private practice as a psychotherapist and clinical supervision consultant. He is the author of a book on clinical supervision in nursing, and numerous journal articles on psychotherapy and

clinical supervision. Stephen is currently undertaking a PhD research study entitled 'A phenomenological study of responses to unrequited love' at the University of Birmingham (UK).

Mic Rafferty RGN, MN, PGCE (FE), Cassel Hospital Certificate in Psychosocial Nursing
Mic was formally Academic Head of Clinical & Professional Development in the School of Health Science, University of Wales, Swansea. Since his retirement Mic continues to be involved on a part-time basis in a range of practice developments and educational courses about clinical supervision. His research interests are about charting the developing meaning of clinical supervision practice and education in West Wales.

Graham Sloan (Clinical Nurse Specialist in Cognitive Behavioural Psychotherapy and Psychosocial Interventions (PSI) for People with Psychosis) PhD BSc (Hons), Dip N (London), Post-Graduate Diploma in Cog Psychotherapy, RMN, RGN
Graham is a Clinical Specialist in Cognitive Psychotherapy and Psychosocial Interventions (PSI) for People with Psychosis, currently working within Consulting and Clinical Psychology Services, NHS Ayrshire & Arran on the Psychosocial Interventions Project and in Adult Psychological Therapy Services. Graham has published widely in the nursing literature and presented at International Conferences. He supervises trainees on the Dundee and South of Scotland Cognitive Therapy courses, clinicians participating in NHS Ayrshire & Arran's PSI course, and qualified CBT specialists pursuing accreditation or who are accredited therapists (consultant clinical psychologists, nurses, and consultant psychiatrists). He is a visiting lecturer at Edinburgh University and Glasgow Caledonian University for Doctorate, MSc in Nursing and BSc (Hons) in Specialist Practice and Community Mental Health Nursing programmes of study. He is an accomplished musician in Jazz, Blues, Rock and Country genres and has a wealth of live performance and recording experience.

Allan Townsend (Psychiatric Nurse Consultant & Teaching Fellow University of Ballarat) Grad Dip. Nursing, BN, RPN, RN
Allan is employed at Ballarat Psychiatric Services (Victoria, Australia) as a Psychiatric Nurse Consultant and is involved in the development and delivery of education for staff, undergraduates and postgraduates. Allan has been instrumental in the development and implementation of clinical supervision in Ballarat and in organizing several clinical supervision conferences in Victoria. Allan has a passion for clinical supervision and an interest in exploring alternative methods of delivery. He is currently involved in trialing the use of videoconferencing between a metropolitan and rural service and has experience of remote clinical supervision on the telephone.

Foreword

The common theme in this thoroughly revised second edition is *engagement* – embracing human encounter through professional conversation between healthcare professionals. It is an ambitious theme, yet one that is appealing to the deeply personal. In this edition, John Driscoll extends an invitation to all healthcare professionals to embrace clinical supervision for their own practice, regardless of their theoretical orientation or the context of their clinical work. He boldly states that clinical supervision is a legitimate practice in healthcare, and has assembled a team of authors with significant expertise from the United Kingdom and Australia, each of whom contribute to the puzzle of clinical supervision, but lessen its mystery by making it more transparent, accessible and do-able. John is well-known in nursing circles for his efforts in promoting the practical aspects of *doing* clinical supervision, implementing clinical supervision, always believing it is possible and believing in its possibilities. The days of 'should we?' or 'shouldn't we?' are well over. Clinical supervision represents 'one of many possibilities for continuing professional development' in health care as a 'legitimate practice-based [form of] learning'.

Not unlike the first edition, this is a book that can be dipped in and out of, depending on the reader's mood and interest. That is the spirit of clinical supervision after all – starting where it feels right at that moment to start, without judgment, just thought and reflection, and there is much to reflect on here. Structurally, the book is divided into four sections, each dealing with specific issues. The eager reader may refer to John and Julia's chapter in Section 1 (The Context of Clinical Supervision) for conceptualizing clinical supervision which, at its heart, concerns reflection, and does not make the usual dichotomy of splitting thinking from feeling. I liked the idea that reflection is 'a work in progress'. Surely this is what we intend when we refer to clinical supervision as forming the basis of the lifelong learner in healthcare practice? The dichotomy, if one must exist, is between the 'challenge and support' aspects of learning. Too much support and one might become disinterested, not learning but turning away, alternatively if there is too much challenge to what one thinks one knows, one might be frightened away. The outcome can be the same. These are delicate matters for considering the engagement made between supervisor and supervisee and there are no hard and fast rules, only a commitment to jointly learn from the clinical supervision experience.

In Section 2 (Getting Going with Clinical Supervision in Practice), Stephen visits the issues of boundaries – of relationship, content, time, space and confidentially; fundamentally the infrastructure of supervision. Without such limits, there can be no safety in supervision and no hope of engagement for either party. For Daniel, engagement in clinical supervision is active, never quite certain, and any successful supervisory partnership requires collaboration and constant attention, perhaps even requiring 'energy and vigour'. Clinical supervision is an active event, and importantly, the imagery used in clinical supervision for reflection is 'something different from our ordinary thinking activities'.

Nevertheless, the book in its entirety threads with its theme of engagement, the idea that clinical supervision is an ordinary human (*albeit* professional) activity, eminently within the reach of everyone who is privileged to work with people within any healthcare organization.

In Section 3 (Supervisory Methods and Approaches), we are treated to two different conceptual frameworks (from psychological counselling) to underpin clinical supervision endeavour. Graham commences his chapter by first pondering his initial and somewhat unsatisfying exposure to clinical supervision where nothing much happened, to later draw out psychological approaches (cognitive-behavioural and solution-focused) that develop a practitioner's therapeutic integrity. Graham reminds us that, in psychological therapies, the patient cannot be understood independently of the therapist, and it is these concerns that necessitate supervision. For some, these are psychoanalytic concepts of transference and counter transference, and for most of us, this is the heart and soul of engaging with others. It is the emotional burden that is so hard to sustain, and there is no doubt that psychological theory is another tool that may help us to stay in there longer with the patient and their suffering. This is the challenge of modern healthcare – to stay with the human, whilst managing the demands of quality service delivery.

Another as yet unexplored theory base to guide supervisory practice, introduced by John and Gerard, is the practice of professional coaching to maximize a supervisees' potential. The links are clear – self-reflection is deceptive, fundamentally so, and having a guide who can see potential and possibility and who is not running the race, so to speak, can offer both an objective perspective and encouragement in healthcare activities being performed. I return to my theme of engagement. For professional growth to occur in us, we need the human, and we need each other. Not just someone who can guide us, but someone who can share the ups and downs, share the emotional burden, and to open our capacity for reflection beyond ourselves, something that is impossible for us to reach on our own.

These are all important functions of clinical supervision, yet in many organizations, engagement in clinical supervision may not be possible due to the tyranny of distance. However the United Kingdom and Australian clinical supervision engagement with this book began initially through the networking between John and Allan via email and telephone, culminating in the first clinical supervision conference held in Ballarat in Victoria in 2003, and then later in Cape Schank in 2005, and outlined in their chapter on Alternative Methods in Clinical Supervision. In this chapter, John and Allan explore how modern technology can bring us physically closer together – an important consideration particularly in a country the size of Australia. Whilst there is nothing new with the continued evolution of technology, what is important is that the element of engagement is possible at all, even without the often preferred face-to-face clinical supervision encounters, in rural and remote healthcare arenas, and present as the only practical option available for professional conversations of this nature.

An increasingly popular approach to practising clinical supervision is in the form of group supervision and is a new chapter to this edition – a forum that undoubtedly offers a form of 'learning from each other'. Many commonly believe that group supervision is more complicated than individual supervision. If there are not group dynamics to consider, as in group therapy, there are developmental stages in the life of the group itself. For the success of the group, John rightly suggests that much rests on the facilitator to steer attention to the group's task of supervision, yet the themes of challenge and support and the process of collaboratively working together – engagement – surface again.

Thus, the scope of this book is grand, but not grandiose, and always with an eye to the practical and the possible, as well as getting things done. How luxurious to simply stop justifying the need for supervision in the healthcare professions, especially nursing.

In Section 4; The Continuing Challenge of Clinical Supervision, John offers his own experiences as an external consultant in implementing clinical supervision throughout a range of healthcare organizations. What will resonate for readers here is that there is no 'right and proper' way of implementation, but rather what is helpful is a 'collaborative style involving honest and constructive conversations' on how to go about getting started. The important thing, as we have come to expect, is engagement.

Finally, Mic, Berwyn and Jeanette invite readers to consider the future practice of clinical supervision. These authors offer us the possibility of well-informed practice standards, based on Proctor's (1986) formative, normative and restorative functions on which to gauge the success (or otherwise) of supervision in practice. Interestingly, they refer to clinical supervision as 'practice supervision', a term adopted in Queensland, Australia, for the health professions, and as a 'medium for the study of relationship dynamics, central to healthcare work'. The circle is complete. We are back to that human, all too human, encounter of engagement.

Finally, I think that if anything will attract healthcare professionals to undertake clinical supervision for their own practice, it is this theme of human engagement. Too often in fast, modern corporations and cost-driven organizations, there is too little thought for the individual and too little time for that human touch. The time spent in clinical supervision awakens that deep yearning for spending moments in thought, in reflection, and in wonder about the work we do with our patients or clients. Clinical supervision is not personal development *per se*, but that human encounter with our patients or clients as they struggle through the healthcare system as we do, affecting the deeply personal in all of us, and we cannot help but be involved, and become *engaged*. Just as clinical supervision is a practice rather more than just a set of skills, there are no 'rules of engagement', there is only engagement. Thank you John and all your authors for sharing your struggles, your triumphs and your hard-won insights and in doing so engaging me in the continued development of clinical supervision.

Tania Yegdich

REFERENCES

Proctor B 1986 Supervision: cooperative exercise in accountability. In: Marken M, Payne M (eds) Enabling and ensuring: supervision in practice. National Youth Bureau, Council for Education and Training in Youth and Community Work, Leicester

Preface

Over a decade has passed since the seeds of clinical supervision were sown into the complex furrows of UK nursing practice as an idea to be developed. Leaning against the metaphorical spade and looking at the growth over this time with the introduction of this second edition aimed not just at nurses but at all healthcare professionals, there have been lots of new shoots, some well-established plants that have since given rise to hybrids, but there remains a lot of weeding, cultivation and nurturing to do if clinical supervision is to survive another decade in healthcare and not wither into the compost of supporting the growth of something else. But that is the normal dynamic nature of growth and change; it requires a lot of hard work, regular effort and commitment for it to be sustained.

I would anticipate that the newer healthcare professions might be able to learn from some of the lessons nursing and health visiting has faced, and continues to face, in the development of clinical supervision. The need for collaboration is plainly evident in an ever-changing and increasingly multiprofessional healthcare environment. I would like to offer this book as a resource in the spirit of that collaboration, in the hope that whatever approach or method you use to develop and practice clinical supervision you will not need to reinvent the wheel, but begin from a place that you know already. Furthermore, I would also urge those same professions not to be coy in coming forward to publish their own, perhaps tentative, clinical supervision experiences so as to establish a collective clinical supervision dialogue among healthcare professionals.

At its simplest, clinical supervision is a regular and formalized reflective conversation between at least two qualified health professionals (although this is fast becoming a remit for all staff), with the intention of both supporting and developing clinical practice. However, within this simplicity lies a complex myriad of choices and challenges, not just for those individuals or groups, but for organizations themselves. With an increased legitimacy for the development of (and evidence of) clinical supervision schemes within the umbrella of healthcare reforms, and specifically clinical governance, clinical supervision is likely to be continually shaped within the tensions of organizational values and cultures, as well as individual health professionals and their own preferences. Within that same hurly-burly of change and reform in healthcare, increased accountability through expanded roles and increased demands for our time, I would suggest, is an urgent need to regularly stop, draw breath and take stock, not just about what we have been doing, but how and why we have been doing it.

Perhaps like the mirror in the bathroom cabinet (or taking it out of a handbag), we are likely to see ourselves as a reflection back, although the intention of using the mirror is usually to improve ourselves, or others (often with a comb or lipstick). Maybe by looking, we may not like what we see, although others might have a different perception, but just doing so from time to time is likely to widen our perceptual field, presenting us with more choices and possibilities than if we had chosen not to.

Some of the most significant issues in the gradual emergence of clinical supervision, for me, since the last edition, have been the obvious mandate that now exists for health professionals to get engaged in the process, the diversity of approaches and the methods being experimented with. These, I suggest, demonstrate a mature growth of clinical supervision, and a movement away from the idea that there is a right and wrong way of going about it. Perhaps readers might think that being reflective, as the subtitle suggests, is a right way of going about clinical supervision. In this respect my views have yet to change from the first edition. While I agree that not all reflection is clinical supervision, I continue to believe that the very act of clinical supervision cannot help but potentiate reflective practice. I say potentiate because, for me, reflective practice remains as just thinking (which is helpful), without some form of action emerging from the encounter.

In this second edition, the overall format has been retained from the original, as the feedback was that it offered a clear structure, and the opportunity to be dipped in and out of, rather than read as a whole. All of the chapters have either been rewritten or are completely new in content, reflecting the progress made since the last edition. On behalf of all the authors, we hope that our commitment and energy for the development of clinical supervision now becomes an inspiration to you, and that you also become part of the ever-increasing critical mass of health professionals who are not just engaging in the process, but actively contributing to its development in whatever healthcare arena they work.

John Driscoll
Professional Development Consultant and Coach
www.supervisionandcoaching.com

Acknowledgements

So many people have been involved, either directly or indirectly, with supporting this second edition. Some who I know are not really that fussed about clinical supervision have been the ones that have shown me the most love and support, and that is of course my wife Anne and Carly and Hayley, my daughters, who resigned themselves to losing me for a significant amount of time and still continue to be bemused at my attempts to facilitate their own reflections. More often than not they, along with Richard and Barbara, offered me their own versions of 'live' supervision and instant feedback on how to balance the hurly-burly of domestic life (including a house move) and co-ordinated the social calendar from their personal perspectives during the life of the project.

My personal thanks go to each of the authors and co-authors for their commitment, dedication and efforts in furthering the cause for the continued development of clinical supervision in international healthcare. In particular, I would like to thank Allan and Daniel for sharing the belief from their side of the world in their chapters, and for inspiring two excellent clinical supervision conferences in 2003 and 2005, which had a direct impact on sowing the seeds for this edition, and clinical supervision generally in Australia. Here's to the next one in Melbourne in 2007! Thank you to Stephen and Graham, who are book authors in their own right, for their continued challenge, support and expertise in clinical supervision. I was so pleased that all the great work that continues in Wales, and in particular the development of standards in clinical supervision, was able to be realized by Mic, Berwyn and Jeanette. A mention here to Steve Cottrell who, along with the late great Georgina Smith, developed such an excellent clinical supervision website resource to share with others from Wales. Special thanks to Julia for agreeing to bring in a physiotherapy as well as an allied health professional perspective to clinical supervision (in among all the other things you were involved in) and to the really supportive library staff at the Chartered Society of Physiotherapy in London. Further thanks to Gerard for opening a door for me into coaching through Noble Manhattan, and your patience as I struggled with making sense and connections with the parallel practice worlds of coaching and clinical supervision. I also need to say a very big thank you here to Rachel who joined me on the journey, and for her own brand of coaching that was enormously helpful and supportive at a time when I was struggling to see any daylight.

My thanks to all those I have had the privilege of co-learning with in supporting clinical supervision efforts in many organizations, but in particular to Ann Girling and Barbara Gaskell, who not just supported but 'appreciated' my efforts in not just thinking about, but then acting on, alternative ways of implementing clinical supervision. To Marcia Hakendorf and Wendy Scott and all the Clinical Supervision Working Party for continuing to support 'appreciative' efforts in implementing clinical supervision in Mental Health Services across South Australia. To Brendan and all the project team of practice developers across the UK for being willing to experiment with the telephone initiative, and in particular to Bob Brown for some great reflections together in Northern Ireland among the black stuff, and to Theresa and Kate from the Foundation of Nursing Studies who supported the book project but probably didn't know it!

Really big thanks for the continued patience and support of Catherine Jackson, Steven Black and Emma Riley, and the professionalism of Elsevier Publishers, Oxford with this edition and for helping me get over the line.

Finally, a sort of thanks to Alfie, my chocolate labrador, for giving me those dreadful doleful eyes while sitting on my feet as I tapped away, and making me get some exercise and a change of scenery from time to time. I am indebted now to your companionship but wasn't always at the time!

Using the book

Throughout the chapters you will meet up with the same (or new) icons from the first edition that are intended to help give you some direction, or simply clarify what you have been reading. Some of them require you to stop and think of the implications of what you have been reading. Often it can be helpful to join up with a colleague or get some peer discussion going to get alternative views of what the icons ask you to do.

THINKING SPACE
This asks you to stop and think for a bit and consider the implications for yourself or your practice.

TIME OUT
This icon is often a 'doing' exercise based on the material within the chapter which you can choose to do alone or with others in your practice area.

HAZARD WARNING
This icon is a warning that what is being described may not be as straightforward as it originally seemed!

HISTORY BOX
These are often personal descriptions or reflections based on the authors' experiences of clinical supervision that serve to illustrate issues going on within the chapter. Often they are accompanied by a reflective dialogue or commentary to help clarify what is happening.

CARTOONS
Throughout the book are some cartoons that serve as metaphors for what is actually trying to be conveyed. You might well still remember significant learning experiences for yourself because they seemed so stupid — and yet you can still remember them a long time after the learning event!

ON REFLECTION
At the end of each chapter appears a bullet-pointed summary of the main chapter content for you to reflect on.

1

THE CONTEXT OF CLINICAL SUPERVISION

1 The place of clinical supervision in modern healthcare

John Driscoll and Julia O'Sullivan

INTRODUCTION

This chapter examines the progression of clinical supervision from being a luxury in healthcare practice, to becoming a central activity in a qualified health professional's continuing professional development legitimized by sweeping modernization reforms, particularly in UK healthcare.

Since the concept of clinical supervision was first introduced into nursing and health visiting over a decade ago, health professionals, other than, but allied to, nursing are now developing workable clinical supervision schemes. It therefore seems an opportune time to collaboratively reflect on what is meant by clinical supervision and some of the lessons being learned through its development.

A distinct advantage of nursing and health visiting having prepared some ground in clinical supervision in terms of organizational infrastructuring through the development of strategies, policies and training is the very real potential for corporate collaboration and sharing of experiences and professional perspectives on clinical supervision.

While for many, clinical supervision in practice is needed, it has also to be valued. An ongoing challenge for the development of formal and planned clinical supervision time for qualified health professionals is not just simply finding the time but convincing them and their managers that engaging in regular clinical supervision can offer significant benefits and is worth supporting in practice.

Not unlike the nursing professions, allied health professions are taking responsibility for the development of clinical supervision and facing the challenges of patient care (rather than staff care) being the priority for practice, whilst wrestling to clarify what is actually meant by clinical supervision, and often with limited resources. Despite these challenges, there undoubtedly is more general awareness of the importance of clinical supervision in healthcare and the development of many different approaches and practices.

In a previous edition, Driscoll (2000:79) outlined a resulting doomsday scenario if nurses and health visitors were not committed to developing workable clinical supervision structures or engaging in the process. Organizations without committed staff were left with three choices. Some of those original organizational choices would now seem more relevant than ever as allied health professionals begin to implement clinical supervision.

- Persevere with the slow uptake of clinical supervision in practice through increased training and continue to 'wait and see'.
- Become disillusioned with the slow uptake and begin to dismantle the clinical supervisory infrastructures that have been put in place.
- Insist that clinical supervision is such a good idea that it is made mandatory for all healthcare practitioners.

While the first option might be the option of choice, it is becoming clear that clinical supervision represents one of many possibilities in satisfying continuing professional development and regulatory needs. It is interesting to note how clinical supervision is increasingly becoming 'less optional' in some organizations as healthcare demands robust auditable structures for staff support and professional development. This is perhaps not surprising with health provision reforming dramatically between inpatient and community provision (Department of Health 2000a, 2004a, 2006) and health professionals' roles expanding rapidly (Department of Health 2006b, Department of Health 2000b, 2003a, Department of Health & Royal College of Nursing 2003) to meet the increase in service-led delivery systems and expectations. In some respects whilst the gradual roll-out of clinical supervision continues and embeds itself into the culture of healthcare organizations, the rapid demands being placed on staff today are even greater and if ever there was a clear mandate for clinical supervision it is now.

One wonders what might be the case if clinical supervision continued to be valued as an auditable mechanism for professional support and development in organizations but remained dormant in health professionals' practice? Might the doomsday scenario (mandatory supervision) then be applied and what might clinical supervision look like then?

As authors, we both remain optimistic that the continued corporate developments in clinical supervision and the good work that has, and continues to be, achieved is now being bolstered by support from the allied health professions. This being the case, we see it as essential that those new to the concept of clinical supervision at least have a working understanding of the concept that will enable them to make some informed choices. In this respect, our intention is that this chapter will demystify clinical supervision and stimulate reflection on what is wanted from clinical supervision and how this can be achieved in practice.

SUPERVISORY STRUCTURES IN HEALTHCARE PRACTICE

Perhaps it is useful to remind oneself that supervision in healthcare is not a new thing although there may well be differences in the emphases or functions of supervision. Therefore, the relationships that occur across the whole spectrum of supervisory activities in the healthcare professions will differ depending on the intentions of those engaging in those processes. For instance, while preceptorship is not an unfamiliar term in nursing and radiography as being a formalized source of support for new professional registrants, in other professions the term mentorship is used. While there are obvious professional nuances, it might be preferable to consider skills and attributes already being used that count as supervisory practice — whether from the perspective of 'supervisor' or 'being supervised'.

Dimensions of supervision

Supervision can be seen as happening in two dimensions (Figure 1.1) and this is a useful way of considering the different types of supervision that are already happening in practice before going on to consider the notion of clinical supervision itself.

Just thinking about the enormous range of supervisory activities gives an indication of the variable nature of the roles of supervisor and supervisee in healthcare and what might be able to be built upon, in terms of the potential development of clinical supervisor and supervisee roles.

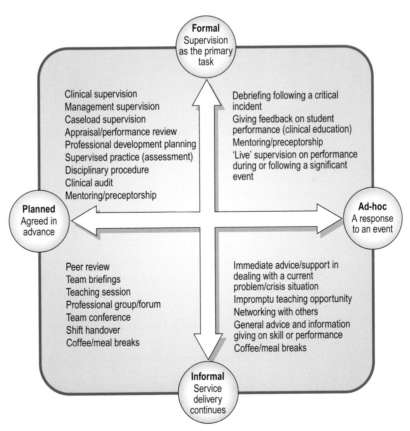

Figure 1.1 Supervisory dimensions already happening in healthcare

Supervisory activities can be said to be two-dimensional, in that they are likely to be 'formal' and 'planned' on the one hand and 'informal' and 'ad-hoc' on the other. The four quadrants in Figure 1.1 relate to the 'where' and 'when' of supervision (and there are likely to be additions from your own experience of supervision). The top right quadrant is particularly useful to consider in adapting supervision activities because it takes into account unexpected happenings in healthcare practice that emerge outside planned supervision times and that may, in themselves, present as more regular supervisory opportunities.

- Compare supervisory activities that already happen in your practice with those in each of the quadrants in Figure 1.1.
- Can you think of any other supervisory practices that might be included in Figure 1.1 based on your own supervisory experiences?

You might be surprised at the amount of supervisory opportunities in clinical practice and perhaps this supports the often stated notion that 'clinical supervision is happening anyway'.

We wonder how many readers would think of the development of clinical supervision as being a 'formal and planned' activity instead of it being a quick-fix solution to an immediate problem in practice. We suggest it might initially be appropriate to make clinical supervision a prominent fixture in practice. Making time for clinical supervision on a par with formal mentoring sessions or monthly team meetings will probably make it more difficult to just 'quietly forget about' it, as these supervisory activities will then be built into the infrastructure of healthcare practice in much the same way as is a medical ward round or case conference.

While clinical supervision may be a new concept to many practitioners, the three main components of supervision in healthcare practice can be summarized as:

- Supervised practice and learning.
- Organizational supervision.
- Supportive supervision.

Supervised practice and learning

We suspect that most readers will have either been through or are going through some form of supervised practice and learning as part of being a health professional. Both parties in this form of supervision–supervisee relationship operate in well-defined roles. The basic parameters include fulfilling institutional, professional and individual learning outcomes as part of a course of pre-qualifying or post-qualifying study. (Confusingly, terms such as clinical education and clinical supervision have often been used interchangeably in this context.) Supervised practice often involves directly instructing or offering advice to the learner as well as having an assessing and supporting function. Mentoring may be considered an example of supervised practice (Higgins & McCarthy 2005) although mentoring functions and roles differ across healthcare disciplines and cultures (Gibson & Heartfield 2005, Morton-Cooper & Palmer 2000:35). Aside from scholarly activities mentoring is also associated with career progression and personal development (Andrews & Wallis 1999, Mills et al 2005) and again cited as clinical supervision (Chow & Suen 2001).

The formal introduction of preceptorship in UK nursing as another form of supervised practice and support was introduced in the 1990s in response to evidence suggesting, rightly, that learning about the newly qualified staff nurse role only really began *after* rather than before qualification (Maben & Macleod-Clark 1996). It has since transformed from being an informal buddying system with a more experienced clinical colleague focusing on skills and role transition in the work setting, to becoming a way of accessing formal support and in-service education for newly qualified staff in practice (CSP 2005a, O'Malley et al 2000).

Supervised practice and learning focuses on the skills and attributes required by an individual to become a newly qualified and accountable health professional but, once that individual becomes qualified, organizational supervision is largely concerned with the maintenance of a professional level of performance. Professional values and organizational expectations of behaviour are defined through the production of formal processes and procedures (such as policies, standards, job descriptors and the joint setting of performance objectives as in appraisal and professional development planning).

- What other examples of organizational supervision are in place for you to adhere to as an individual practitioner?
- How are you involved in ensuring that such organizational supervision structures are working in practice with other staff ... what is your contribution?
- How are organizational structures of supervision similar to or different from supervised practice and learning methods?

The focus of organizational or managerial forms of supervision is on the performance of the individual or group of individuals in the wider organization.

You will not be surprised to discover that this type of supervision is traditionally thought of as a form of employer surveillance. While that statement might be a generalization, there is undoubtedly a tendency in this form of supervision towards managing risk and setting goals and objectives based on corporate strategies. The notion of surveillance is only confirmed when these strategies cover areas of disciplinary procedure. However, this type of supervision is not unusual; some junior health professionals in, for example, physiotherapy and occupational therapy are rotated through departments in which supervision by a more senior member of staff is expected. Therefore, perhaps, it is not difficult to see how suspicion can be aroused when the term supervision is used in practice.

Supportive supervision

Perhaps as a consequence of heavy-handed supervision experiences, and in order to survive the rigours of clinical practice, health professionals have always created individualized support systems at work. (You may wish to compare again the different types of support in Figure 1.1 with your own practice.) Some emerge almost intuitively, from working with and knowing that you can trust particular people who are prepared to listen to your concerns. Butterworth (1998:8) describes, as an example of informal peer support, the 'tea break / tear break' used by nurses as a way of letting colleagues share in the stressful clinical experiences which had affected their working day. Such ad-hoc and informal encounters play a vital part in coping with everyday clinical practice. While not exactly clinical supervision, such support networks can be considered the cement that holds the building up, without which it might implode!

We wonder, for health professionals who do not have a booked diary of patients, if reinstating formalized dinner breaks, based away from clinical areas, might offer opportunities for supportive supervision and reduce professional isolation (as opposed to grabbing a sandwich and sitting alone in the busy work environment). This is not to say that every lunch break should constitute clinical supervision, but by meeting regularly to discuss work, away from the workplace, opportunities could be created for the provision of any support that might be needed.

The changing face of healthcare practice so vividly described by Ferguson (2005:293) clearly endorses the need for formal as well as informal supportive supervision mechanisms in practice:

> ... Health services have been integrated into the community, and the professionals that remain in 'traditional' institutions experience a much changed landscape. Staff numbers have reduced, middle management has been downsized and, information technology and flexible work practices bring an unfamiliar isolation for the health worker. The needs of the individual health professional now, more than ever before need urgent attention ...

Looking at the range of supervision schemes in Figure 1.1:
a) In what dimensions do you give supervision and for what reasons?
b) In what dimensions do you receive supervision (if at all), and for what reasons?
c) In what ways might supportive supervision differ from other forms of supervision that occur in your practice area?
d) What evidence is there to support, or refute, the notion that supportive supervision is happening already in your practice area?

Morton-Cooper and Palmer (2000:209) provide a much needed graphic representation that we have adapted to help summarize the range of supervision schemes, outlined previously, that would likely be encountered in becoming and being a healthcare professional (Figure 1.2).

In times of change and challenge in healthcare practice it is normal for practitioners to feel uncertain and confused. It is also normal, in our view, to expect organizations to provide and actively develop the shaping of workable and supportive supervision schemes that are, in turn, actively utilized by practitioners. So, as there is already a range of supervisory structures in healthcare practice, why the emergence of another supervisory structure called clinical supervision?

THE EMERGENCE OF CLINICAL SUPERVISION IN HEALTHCARE SETTINGS

Not unlike other supervisory processes, clinical supervision is a particular kind of professional conversation that happens in the workplace. But, unlike some of those other supervisory processes, clinical supervision sets out not to be the kind of conversation that involves giving people advice, assessing them or solving their problems for them, but one in which you provide space, time and professional

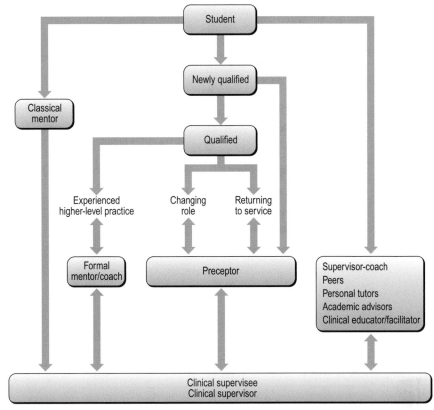

Figure 1.2 The range and significance of supervision schemes in healthcare practice

support for colleagues to reflect on their encounters with patients or fellow workers (Burton & Launer 2003a).

As a means of professional learning and support, clinical supervision is not a new idea within certain health and social care professions, for example:

■ social work (Browne & Bourne 1996, Kadushin & Harkness 2002, Morrison 2003),

■ counselling and psychotherapy (Hawkins & Shohet 2000, Haynes et al 2003, Hughes & Pengelly 1997, Page & Wosket 2002, Tudor & Worrall 2004),

■ midwifery (Kirkham 1996, Nursing & Midwifery Council 2005a, Skoberne 2003, Thomas 2005),

■ mental health professionals (Ask & Roche 2005, NMAG 2004, Scaife 2002),

■ occupational therapy (COT 1997, Hall 1998, Sweeney et al 2001),

■ speech and language therapy (RCSLT 1996), and

■ some nursing specialities (Butterworth et al 1998, Cutcliffe et al 2001).

Not surprisingly much of the current literature on the development of clinical supervision for nurses and allied health professionals, particularly in the UK, has emerged from these professional disciplines where supervision has already become an integral part of clinical practice and often a mandatory accreditation requirement.

For other health-related disciplines, clinical supervision is just beginning to emerge in practice, for example:

- dietetics (Burton 2000, Kirk et al 2000),
- the medical profession (Burton & Launer 2003b:3, Grant et al 2003, McDonald 2002),
- occupational health (Billington et al 2005),
- physiotherapy (CSP 2005b, Clouder & Sellars 2004, Sellars 2000),
- podiatry (Weaver 2001),
- radiography (Hussain 2004, Sood & Driscoll 2004),
- learning disabilities nursing (Malin 2000),
- practice nursing (Cheater & Hale 2001, Cutcliffe & McFeely, 2001, Debreczeny 2003, Greaves 2004),
- complementary therapies (Ryan 2004, Tate et al 2003, Wood 2003), and
- prison nursing (Freshwater et al 2001, 2002).

More detailed reviews about the emergence of clinical supervision can be found in:

- Grover (2002), Grauel (2002), Hunter and Blair (1999), McMahon and Patton (2002), Rose and Best (2005) and Sellars (2004) for allied health professionals,
- Kilminster and Jolly (2000) for medical staff, and
- Bond and Holland (1998), Cutcliffe and Lowe (2005), Fowler (1996), Gilmore (2001), Hyrkas et al (1999), Stevenson (2005), Winstanley and White (2003) and Yegdich (2002) for nursing.

From our experience in facilitating workshops, the term 'supervision' when applied to healthcare practice, whether for senior qualified practitioners or student learners, still manages to conjure up images of being 'watched' or 'controlled' in some way by those responsible for the overall management of the service delivery. This is despite the efforts made to dissociate the continuing professional development and more supportive mechanism of clinical supervision for qualified clinical staff from more organizationally led models of supervision such as appraisal, individual performance reviews and caseload management. Yegdich and Cushing (1998) go further and suggest that in nursing a name change is needed because while the need for clinical supervision is largely unquestioned, and it is viewed as a 'good thing', its implementation, particularly in nursing, has been slow and tortuous and met with scepticism, ridicule and resistance and this remains a cause for concern (Cottrell 2002, Yegdich 2002:251).

- What does the term 'clinical supervision' mean for you as a qualified healthcare professional?
- Does the term 'clinical supervision' seem to reflect what is expected to happen?
- Do you think a name change would increase the uptake of clinical supervision by healthcare professionals?
- What might be an alternative term(s) for best describing what happens in clinical supervision?

Since clinical supervision, as a term, has such a poor reputation why not simply change its name, as Yegdich and Cushing (1998) suggest, and thus change its standing in the healthcare community? Unfortunately, clinical supervision has already many names, being described interchangeably as:

- a form of critical companionship, being a metaphor for a person-centred helping relationship for facilitating emancipatory learning experiences in practice (Manley et al 2005, Titchen 2003),
- clinical facilitation (Lambert & Glacken 2005),
- clinical education (Sellars 2004),
- development coaching (Driscoll & Cooper 2005),
- guided reflection (Johns 2000, Todd & Freshwater 1999), or simply
- professional supervision (Ferguson 2005), among others.

However, this proliferation of terms indicates that professionals in healthcare see that struggling with the concept of clinical supervision is worthwhile. For example, at an Egalitarian Consultation Meeting (ECM) considering multiprofessional clinical supervision in mental health, participants were given the task of constructing their own particular version of clinical supervision (as an alternative to the received wisdom that there is only one right way); time and space were deliberately set aside during the meeting for the accomplishment of the task (Stevenson 2005, Stevenson & Jackson 2000).

Clearly there is a need for a diversity of clinical supervision approaches as the original idea of a 'one fit all' approach has become outdated. Our own appreciation and experiences of clinical supervision suggest that there is a need to continue to promote a *clinical 'soup' ervision* and experiment with eclectic blends to validate whether or not they are useful processes for practitioners engaging in clinical supervision. However, as Power (1999:11) warns:

> ... the real problem is that the more words we use to avoid the ones that we have — and should be using (clinical supervision) — the more we dig a bigger hole for ourselves ...

It is perhaps reassuring to note that confusion often experienced by introducing the term 'clinical supervision' to practitioners in UK healthcare would seem to be not only a national but also an international issue. For instance, clinical supervision relates to the supervised practice of nursing students on clinical placements in Canada and New Zealand (Mills et al 2005, Rose & Best 2005), and is a term that has been used interchangeably with managerial supervision and supervised practice in nursing in Australia (Winstanley & White 2003, Yegdich & Cushing 1998) until quite recently.

Cutcliffe and Lowe (2005) also cite significant differences in the perception of the purpose of clinical supervision when comparing North American and European conceptualizations.

- In North America, clinical supervisors are seen as being clinical experts in a given speciality and often have a managerial role.
- In Europe, rather than being thought of as clinical experts, clinical supervisors might be peers and be expected to be supportive at facilitating reflective practice and helping the supervisee solve practice difficulties.

- The latter approach has also been significant in the development of clinical supervision in Scandinavia (Hyrkas 2005, Hyrkas et al 1999, Palsson & Norberg 1995, Paunonen & Hyrkas 2001, Severinsson & Hallberg 1996).

Whatever the international differences, the profile of clinical supervision in UK healthcare is undoubtedly being shaped both by governmental policy and professional ideas about its development. These two influences create a dynamic tension affecting its implementation because of the differences in managerial and professional agendas; the former being concerned with developing a safe and accountable health professional, the latter more concerned with continued personal learning and support. Although Malin (2000) questions whose interests are best being served, both agendas appear to have a place in describing the overall functions of clinical supervision and are discussed in more detail in the next section.

Clinical governance, a central plank in governmental healthcare reforms, is a statutory quality framework through which all NHS organizations are accountable for continually improving the quality of their services (Department of Health 1999, 1998a, 1998b, NHSCGST 2005, McSherry & Pearce 2002, Scally & Donaldson 1998). It has dramatically raised the profile of continuing professional development (CPD) and work-based learning initiatives because its statutory professional regulations must be met (Butterworth & Woods 1999, CSP 2005b, Gustafsson & Fagerberg 2004, NMC 2005b).

Thus the demand for accountability has highlighted the role of clinical supervision in the process of expanding professional roles and change and reform in healthcare (Department of Health 2006b, Department of Health 2000b, 2000c, 2000d, 2003a, Department of Health & Royal College of Nursing 2003, Sellars 2004). More recently, healthcare organizations have had to demonstrate that they have staff support structures in place, such as clinical supervision, as they have become auditable mechanisms within the NHS (CHAI 2004) and have spawned a number of multiprofessional organizational policies on clinical supervision (Clough et al 2005, Harder et al 2005).

Although clinical supervision is not mandatory for most UK health professionals, it is viewed as best practice; to the point that it is fast becoming a 'must do' in healthcare organizations as a method of ongoing staff development. Also, with the revised pay and conditions now including supervision in job descriptions and supervision generally becoming a core dimension of the Knowledge and Skills Framework for continued career progression (Department of Health 2003b, 2004b, Royal College of Nursing 2005), its importance is acknowledged.

A recent lengthy consultation of allied health professions endorsed clinical supervision as a legitimate form of continuing professional development (HPC 2004, 2005) and a number of professional bodies have developed specific clinical supervision frameworks (BDA 2000, COT 1997, CSP 2005b, SCoR 2003a, 2003b, RCSLT 1996).

While clinical supervision has become a more visible concept, one wonders who will be responsible for the policing and development of 'less optional', if not quite mandatory, clinical supervision schemes in practice. It could be argued that the development of clinical supervision schemes might be easier to implement in organizations that view them as not 'optional' but necessary and who set about formalizing frameworks and policies. However, Edwards et al (2005) remain sceptical and posit that, despite these measures, the actual finding of the time and resources to implement such schemes will remain an ongoing issue. In addition, what of those health professionals who simply choose not to engage in clinical supervision where it is not a definite professional requirement but rather seen as just 'best practice'?

Despite some very real challenges associated with the concept of clinical supervision, there seems to be some consensus of opinion about the ingredients of the clinical supervision encounter:

- managerial elements,
- personal support elements, and
- learning elements.

The current debate is around the proportions of each of these elements that one must include to distinguish supervision from managerial interventions, from learning and from therapy *per se*, or more specifically to fully understand the purpose and functions of clinical supervision in practice.

THE PURPOSE AND FUNCTIONS OF CLINICAL SUPERVISION

The importance of taking regular time out to talk about practice is a key consideration in clinical supervision and a consistent feature of working definitions of clinical supervision from the literature, for instance:

> ... a structured, formal process that enables dieticians to discuss their work with an experienced practitioner, trained to facilitate clinical supervision. This discussion should be a guided reflection on current practice and should be used to learn from experience ...
> BDA (British Dietetic Association), 2000

> ... an exchange between practicing professionals to assist the development of professional skills.
> Butterworth, 1992:12

Talking about clinical practice in clinical supervision also provides a learning opportunity and a way of influencing change in future practice(s):

> ... an opportunity for a professional to change a story about a working encounter by holding a conversation with another professional.
> Launer, 2003:94

While regularly talking about practice is a key consideration in clinical supervision, unless it is properly formalized and legitimized as a practice-based activity (as important as working with clients and patients), it will continue to be difficult to implement. This aspect is discussed further in Chapter 9. Actively finding the time, in among all of the pressures that exist at work, demonstrates not only a commitment to the process of clinical supervision, whether as a supervisor or supervisee, but also values the importance of taking time for yourself while you continue to care for others.

- What difference do you think it would make in clinical practice to make time to formally stop and discuss your work with someone you have confidence in on a regular basis?
- What might be the implications of NOT doing so for:
  a) yourself?
  b) your colleagues?
  c) your patients/clients?
  d) your organization?
  e) your family and friends?

The plethora of definitions of clinical supervision in the literature raises, perhaps unrealistic, expectations about the effectiveness of the process for both practitioners and their practice. For instance, along with definitions previously cited in this chapter, they include the following premises (or are they promises?):

- a process for maintaining and safeguarding standards of care in practice;

- being evidence of lifelong learning in practice;

- a recognition of individual practitioner responsibilities and accountabilities under clinical governance;

- contributing to significant improvement in healthcare delivery through regular reflection on practice with others;

- a process for the development of practitioner knowledge and subsequent increased professional skills and competence;

- a method of practice-based learning contributing to the continuing professional development of the practitioner;

- a formal method of support to influence personal change in order to improve future practice.

You may be able to think of other reasons why effective clinical supervision raises the expectations for practice. But, none the less, these expectations could be utilized by clinical supervisors to encourage the development of competence in practitioners as well as themselves.

It is important to begin to think of clinical supervision not only in terms of individual outcomes for healthcare professionals, but also as a way of improving the quality of healthcare delivery. A popular and well thought out UK nursing definition proposed by Bond and Holland (1998:12) continues to offer not just the 'what' but 'why' of clinical supervision and would seem to encompass many of the principles enshrined in definitions of clinical supervision:

Clinical supervision is regular protected time for facilitated, in-depth reflection on clinical practice. It aims to enable the supervisee to achieve, sustain and creatively develop a high quality of practice through the means of focused support and development. The supervisee reflects on the part she plays as an individual in the complexities of the events and the quality of her practice. This reflection is facilitated by one or more experienced colleagues who have expertise in facilitation and the frequent on-going sessions are led by the supervisee's agenda. The process of clinical supervision should continue throughout the person's career, whether they remain in clinical practice or move into management, research or education.

While definitions can offer substance to a rather nebulous concept like clinical supervision it is unlikely that one definition will be able to capture all the complexities of healthcare practice. However, having in the back of your mind the 'what' and 'why' of clinical supervision can be helpful when trying to explain to colleagues what it is and what it sets out to do. (This is particularly relevant when those colleagues are covering for you in your practice.)

- If you are new to clinical supervision, whether as a clinical supervisor or supervisee, read over Bond and Holland's definition (or your own professional or organizational definition) and write down what for you constitutes:
  - the functions (the 'what') of clinical supervision;
  - the purpose of (the 'why') of clinical supervision.
- If you are an experienced clinical supervisor or supervisee you may wish to read over Bond and Holland's definition and compare this to your current experiences in clinical supervision. How does it match up to what you are doing already or what might need to alter?
- How does the definition help you in articulating the 'what' and the 'why' of clinical supervision to peer colleagues?

While self-reported practitioner outcomes may not be that difficult to evaluate, improvements in patient/client outcomes remain the 'holy grail' for clinical supervision and will continue to be a major challenge because of the multitude of other variables that prevail or have an effect on multiprofessional healthcare delivery. However, organizational data exist that might be correlated with the onset of clinical supervision. For instance, Brigid Proctor's (1986) Interactive Framework of Clinical Supervision is currently one of the most widely used clinical supervision frameworks, particularly in nursing practice (Sloan & Watson 2002, Winstanley & White 2003). The framework, based on an original framework by Kadushin (1992), has since formed the basis for a number of evaluations in practice (Butterworth et al 1997, Bowles & Young 1999) and a national audit tool for measuring the effectiveness of clinical supervision in organizations, the Manchester Clinical Supervision Scale (Winstanley 2000), and has been influential in the development of standards in clinical supervision across Wales (Rafferty et al 2003), which is outlined in more detail in Chapter 10.

The three interactive functions of clinical supervision (Figure 1.3) present a practical framework that we have used in training clinical supervisors. It offers at least three different perspectives or foci and can be used as an aide when the supervisee is preparing for a clinical supervision discussion.

Referring back to Bond and Holland's (1998) definition, it is also possible to see how Proctor's functions of clinical supervision might relate to each other in practice. It is interesting to speculate that clinical supervisors may have preferred functions or styles that they use in clinical supervision. For example:

- for practitioners who have an unavoidable dual function, being both a clinical supervisor and manager of a supervisee, the normative element may be a more natural function to use during a supervisory discussion;

- someone working in a mental health setting might adopt more of a supportive function; or

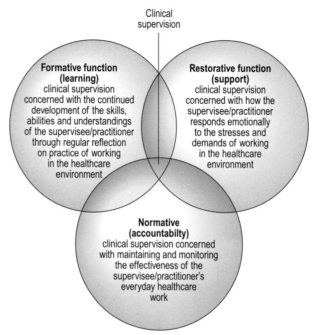

Figure 1.3 Three functions of Proctor's interactive model

- a clinical education facilitator acting as a clinical supervisor might adopt more of a learning function.

The three elements or functions of clinical supervision were always intended to be applied equally, but in reality they tend to overlap or compete because supervisees often present with a complexity of issues. A clinical supervision model cannot be applied too rigidly; it has to be a flexible tool that can initiate or guide clinical supervision.

- If you are already an active clinical supervisor do you have a preferred supervisory function and what might be the implications of this for your supervisee?
- Do you think it should be the supervisee or the supervisor that determines which of Proctor's functions takes priority in the clinical supervision discussion? What factors would help you come to a decision?
- Might it be possible to use all three of Proctor's functions in a clinical supervision discussion and what might be the implications of this?

Although Proctor's framework is a useful tool for conceptualizing supervision by breaking it into component parts, like most models, it is an artificial construct that is unlikely to totally reflect reality. It might therefore be considered a useful but limited guide that cannot be expected to cover every eventuality.

It is our contention that Proctor's framework is a useful beginner's guide to clinical supervision and that practitioners may then wish to progress or experiment with other supervision frameworks as the supervisor and supervisee become more confident in the supervisory relationship and more open to exploring other perspectives. For example, in Proctor's framework there is not a function specifically examining the relationship of the supervisee to a patient/client, whereas in some psychological-based frameworks this perspective is prominent. (This is dealt with in more detail in Chapter 5.)

An example from Sood and Driscoll (2004) of the discussions in clinical supervision using Proctor's framework is summarized in Box 1.1.

BOX 1.1	*A summary of Proctor's supervisory functions in relation to what a supervisee discussed in clinical supervision (Sood & Driscoll 2004)*

FORMATIVE FUNCTION (learning)

■ How to be a supervisee and get the most from sessions

■ Articulating what clinical supervision is to others

■ Writing as well as talking about practice

■ Use of a structured framework to help with reflection on practice

■ Being more assertive in practice

■ Use of own experiential learning to develop further knowledge about being a carer within a family and increased awareness of patient/client needs

■ The importance of networking in a post that is often isolated from immediate peers (i.e. other Macmillan radiographers)

■ Development of a deeper insight of the impact of self on others at work

RESTORATIVE FUNCTION (support)

■ The dangers of becoming too involved with caseloads to see objectively

■ Personal feelings that can surface from everyday working with the patient/client and their family

■ Personal effects of trying to be all things to all people in the caring situation

■ The need to recognize as well as establish a support network in the immediate work environment to survive the stresses and strains of working in oncology

■ Giving oneself (and actively seeking) permission to take time out on a regular basis to reflect on practice with someone outside of practice

NORMATIVE (accountability)

■ Examining how a 'small fish' swims in a big pond

■ Roles and responsibilities in practice

■ Clarification of role boundaries in practice

■ Establishing the legitimacy of clinical supervision by 'finding the time' in busy practice

■ Less defensive and more open about strengths and limitations in own practice

■ Questioning own leadership potential

WHAT ARE YOUR EXPECTATIONS FOR ENGAGING IN CLINICAL SUPERVISION?

To make more informed decisions on how the process of clinical supervision can be incorporated into everyday healthcare practice, we think it is important to have explored the background to its emergence and the different agendas and expectations that come with such an initiative. Looking back over what has been discussed in this chapter, you might feel that the emphasis has largely been on identifying what clinical supervision may or may not be, according to other people's ideas — people who think they know about you and your practice (perhaps including us!).

- In what ways are other people's agendas for implementing clinical supervision similar to, or different from, your own?
- What might be the consequences of that for you and your practice?
- What do you consider to be the distinguishing features of clinical supervision so that others might be able to recognize it in practice?

You may wish to compare your thoughts with some of ours contained in Box 1.2 (not in any order of priority). These ideas will be further expanded in Chapters 3 and 4.

BOX 1.2	*Some distinguishing features of clinical supervision in practice*

- A confidential process (with exceptions) in which a supervisee practitioner discloses significant aspects of their practice to a chosen clinical supervisor (who may or may not be from the same healthcare discipline)
- A planned and intentional opportunity to talk, within previously agreed boundaries, about practice
- Involves a clinical supervisor and supervisee practitioner (or group of practitioners) reflecting openly on practice with the intention of improving care delivery
- An expectation that clinical supervisors will have had some form of training to be able to facilitate effective clinical supervision in others as well as being in regular clinical supervision themselves
- A regular process of support reinforced by the healthcare organization that is in addition to those informal support mechanisms already existing in practice
- A practice-based form of learning, the evidence of which can contribute towards meeting continuing professional development (CPD) requirements
- An additional process in practice that is distinct from formal line management supervision structures, although it is acknowledged that a dual role might co-exist
- The meeting moves from simply talking about practice to working towards some demonstrable actions or a changed perspective on the supervisee's practice
- The process supports positive challenging by both parties in clinical supervision
- There is unlikely to be one single model that will suit all practitioners, so flexibility is required in the supervisory approach taken

As you will have already noted, the push towards the implementation of clinical supervision is being driven by:

■ healthcare reforms,

■ structural changes in that provision,

■ public concerns about education and clinical practice, and

■ an overdue recognition of the need for active support in practice.

Again, you may feel that clinical supervision is being developed, or simply wished for, by those who are at arm's length from the reality of everyday practice.

While facilitating clinical supervision workshops, we have been interested to note how different clinical supervision appears to be when looked at from different points of view. For example:

■ a newly qualified occupational therapist who is wanting information on what is expected of them as a supervisee,

■ a superintendent physiotherapist in a primary care trust who will be managing the initiative in clinical practice, or

■ an executive director seeking ways of maximizing the resources being set aside for its development in line with clinical governance.

Whatever the perspective, for clinical supervision to continue to be sustained in everyday healthcare practice it must have some demonstrable outcomes, not just for the practitioner (perhaps as professional development), but, more importantly, for practice (by the way that care is delivered through development and improvement).

To improve your clinical supervisory techniques, you have to engage regularly in actual clinical supervision activities. Thus, by regular participation, you develop, through your own supervisory experience(s), a method and format that works for you. In other words, you are able to apply a way of engaging in clinical supervision that makes sense not just to the supervisor, but to the supervisee and, just as importantly, through such commitment and effort, makes an impact on practice.

Perhaps a starting point for your own reflections, or even getting started in clinical supervision, might be to consider how participating in clinical supervision could contribute beneficially to your practice.

Many of the benefits described in the evaluative literature have a tendency to report on outcomes for practitioners themselves rather than for patients/clients.

There still exist unanswered questions about organizations continuing to invest in the development of clinical supervision without also having some form of demonstrable return in relation to users of the health services (Edwards et al 2005). Interestingly this would seem to be a topical issue for a discipline like psychotherapy where regular supervision has already beeen an integral part of practice and training for many years (Bambling 2004).

However, Debreczeny (2003:76) argues that if healthcare professionals are more confident and capable in the work setting then professional practice will be improved and patients/clients will benefit. Ongoing research continues to be concerned with these issues.

In what ways do you think that committing to regular clinical supervision in practice offers benefits to:
a) yourself as a practitioner?
b) the people you deliver a professional healthcare service to?
c) the organization that employs you to deliver that service?

Some of the broad benefits cited for engaging in regular clinical supervision in nursing have been (Butterworth et al 1997, Cheater & Hale 2001, Hyrkas 2005, Severinsson & Borgenhammar 1997, Teasdale et al 2001):

■ increased feelings of support,

■ reductions in professional isolation,

■ reductions in levels of stress,

■ reductions in emotional exhaustion and burnout

■ increased job satisfaction and morale.

Current research and evaluations being carried out within the allied health professions in healthcare on the benefits of clinical supervision also highlight a similar range of positive outcomes (Grover 2002, Sellars 2000, 2004, Strong et al 2003, Tate et al 2003, Weaver 2001). Strong et al (2003) classified the following themes as important benefits in the supervisory practice of allied health professionals in a mental health service that also seem to resonate as functions of clinical supervision previously outlined by Proctor (1986):

■ Professional development and support in practice.

■ A method of quality assurance and competent best practice.

■ Support for organizational issues such as recruitment and retention.

■ Increased professional discipline growth and identity.

■ Promotion of work-based learning and the development of new skills.

An important issue in much of the evaluative literature on clinical supervision is the centrality of the supervisory relationship (see also Chapter 4) as supporting positive outcomes, while ineffective clinical supervision can exacerbate increased job dissatisfaction (Hyrkas 2005, Schroffel 1999), and has obvious implications for its continued development.

Clearly, for clinical supervision to become fully integrated into everyday clinical practice, it first requires health professionals to have a dialogue in order to come to a shared understanding of:

■ what is wanted,

■ what the key features of it are when compared to other forms of supervision that already exist, and

■ how to move from being something 'extra' ordinary in practice to something more ordinary.

In many cases, in our view, this involves examining the structures that already exist and how they can be adapted for use in clinical supervision practice.

CONCLUSION

It would seem that the debate about the place of clinical supervision for health professions in modern healthcare is clearly well advanced in some disciplines while for others it is just beginning. In the expansion of professional roles in the modernization of services through policy directives, it is possible to see a blurring of professional boundaries in which the development of collaborative supervision schemes (Clough 2005, Harder et al 2005) and training may well become the norm. Although perhaps a challenge at the outset, it does seem not only increasingly likely but also a common-sense (as well as cost-efficient) way forward — as opposed to individual disciplines scrapping for limited resources and developing their own schemes within the same healthcare organizations.

The professional agenda does include a compelling argument for all practitioners to now have access to clinical supervision whether mandatory, non-optional or statutory. The key, as always, is in the detail, in which the weighting for the range of different intentions and purposes surrounding clinical supervision still requires some clarification. One framework will not fit all, but a range of methods and formats should be available and agreed on at the local level.

The time has come to encourage practitioners to develop a form of clinical supervision that will meet their individual needs, by simply starting regular professional conversations in practice. Through these conversations, supervisees will be able to process the personal experiences they are struggling with rather than focus on the policies or procedures that others perceive as important. In other words, practitioners should be actively supported to challenge the received wisdom of those who think they know what 'should' happen in clinical supervision.

While this chapter has been an attempt to offer an overview of the development of clinical supervision, it has also tried to demystify and debunk some of the myths that still surround it and impede its continued development. It might be argued that the bar for the organizational development of clinical supervision has been raised so high as to now have become a universal remedy for all the challenges in modernizing professional healthcare rather than a practice improvement potential. Perhaps when all the hype is stripped away from the veneer of clinical supervision we are left with what Darley (2001) refers to as:

> ... a useful if rather dull process whereby practitioners are listened to by someone who has the ability (organizationally, interpersonally or professionally) to help them ... help in this context means to resolve any concerns they may have with their work and to help develop their practice by a process of guided reflection ...

A legitimate opportunity remains and it is now up to healthcare professionals to collectively shape what they themselves consider to be clinical supervision before it becomes shaped by others on their behalf.

On reflection . . . chapter summary

- Supervision in professional healthcare is not a new concept although there are differences in emphases and functions in clinical practice.
- Clinical supervision can be viewed as a regular professional conversation in practice for practice.
- There is a need for a diversity of approaches in clinical supervision, as a 'one fit all' approach has become outdated.
- Clinical supervision has now become a legitimate practice-based learning activity supporting individual practitioners' continuing professional development.
- While not mandatory for most health professionals, clinical supervision is now becoming 'less optional' in clinical practice.
- For clinical supervision to flourish in practice and justify resources it must have some demonstrable outcomes not just for the practitioner, but the way care is delivered to service users.
- The supervisory relationship is a key feature in supporting positive outcomes of clinical supervision.
- Clinical supervision may now have become a universal remedy for all the challenges in modernizing professional healthcare.

REFERENCES

Andrews M, Wallis M 1999 Mentorship in nursing: a literature review. Journal of Advanced Nursing 29(1):201–207

Ask A, Roche A 2005 Clinical supervision: a practical guide for the alcohol and other drugs field. National Centre for Education and Training on Addition (NCETA) and Flinders University, Adelaide, Australia

Bambling M 2004 The developmental model of supervision in contemporary practice. Psychotherapy in Australia 11(1):30–35

BDA 2000 Guidance document clinical supervision for dieticians. The British Dietetic Association (Dieticians). Online. Available: http://members.bda.uk.com/Downloads/clinsuperdiet.pdf. Accessed 12/10/05

Billington D, Hallinan C, Robinson A 2005 Propelling towards professional supervision. Occupational Health 57(2):24–28

Bond M, Holland S 1998 Skills of clinical supervision for nurses. Open University, Milton Keynes, UK

Bowles N, Young C 1999 An evaluative study of clinical supervision based on Proctor's three function interactive model. Journal of Advanced Nursing 30(4):958–964

Browne A, Bourne I 1996 The social work supervisor. Open University Press, Buckinghamshire, UK

Burton J, Launer J 2003a Primary care and the need for clinical supervision and support. In: Burton J, Launer J 2003 (eds) Supervision and support in primary care. Radcliffe Medical Press, Oxford, UK, p 3–14

Burton J, Launer J (eds) 2003b Supervision and support in primary care. Radcliffe Medical, Oxford, UK

Burton S 2000 A critical essay on professional development in dietetics through a process of reflection and clinical supervision. Journal of Human Nutrition and Dietetics (5):317–322

Butterworth T 1992 Clinical supervision as an emerging idea in nursing. In: Butterworth T, Faugier J (eds) Clinical supervision and mentorship in nursing. Chapman & Hall, London, p 3–17

Butterworth T 1998 Clinical supervision as an emerging idea in nursing. In: Butterworth T, Faugier J, Burnard P (eds) Clinical supervision and mentorship in nursing. 2nd edn. Stanley Thornes, Cheltenham, UK, p 1–18

Butterworth T, Carson J, White E et al 1997 It is good to talk. An evaluation study in England and Scotland. The School of Nursing, Midwifery and Health Visiting, University of Manchester, Manchester, UK

Butterworth T, Faugier J, Burnard P (eds) 1998 Clinical supervision and mentorship in nursing. 2nd edn. Stanley Thornes, Cheltenham, UK

Butterworth T, Woods D 1999 Clinical supervision and clinical governance: working together to ensure safe and accountable practice. University of Manchester, Manchester, UK

CHAI 2004 Cambridgeshire and Peterborough mental health partnership NHS trust clinical governance review (may) commission for healthcare audit and inspection. Online. Available: www.chai.org.uk/assetRoot/04/00/17/56/0 4001756.pdf. Accessed 18/09/05

Cheater F, Hale C 2001 An evaluation of a local clinical supervision scheme for practice nurses. Journal of Clinical Nursing 10(1):119–131

Chow F, Suen L 2001 Clinical staff as mentors in pre-registration undergraduate nursing education: students' perceptions of the mentors' roles and responsibilities. Nurse Education Today 21:350–358

Clouder L, Sellars J 2004 Reflective practice and clinical supervision: an interprofessional perspective. Journal of Advanced Nursing 46(3):262–269

Clough A 2005 Nursing and allied health professional strategy 2005–2007 (Theme 6.5:2) Clinical Quality. Online. Available: http://www.salford-pct.nhs.uk/ board_reports/board_reports_200105/ Nursing%20Strategy%20- %20Agenda%20Item%20No%207.pdf#se arch='meeting%20the%20challenge%20al lied%20health%20professionals%20NHS. Accessed 25/10/05

COT (1997) Statement on supervision of occupational therapy. College of Occupational Therapy, London

Cottrell S 2002 Suspicion, resistance, tokenism and mutiny: problematic dynamics relevant to the implementation of clinical supervision in nursing. Journal of Psychiatric and Mental Health Nursing 9:667–671

CSP 2005a Guidelines of good practice for new entrants (CPD Information Paper CPD 2). The Chartered Society of Physiotherapy, London

CSP 2005b A Guide to implementing clinical supervision (Information Paper: CPD 37). The Chartered Society of Physiotherapy, London

Cutcliffe J, Butterworth T, Proctor B (eds) 2001 Fundamental themes in clinical supervision. Routledge, London

Cutcliffe J, Lowe L 2005 A comparison of North American and European conceptualizations of clinical supervision. Issues in Mental Health Nursing 26:475–488

Cutcliffe J, McFeely S 2001 Practice nurses and their lived experience of clinical supervision. British Journal of Nursing 10(5):312–323

Darley G 2001 Demystifying supervision. Nursing Management 7(10):18–21

Debreczeny S 2003 Nursing supervision in primary care. In: Burton J, Launer J (eds) Supervision and support in primary care. Radcliffe Medical, Oxford, UK, p 67–77

Department of Health 1998a A first class service – quality in the new NHS. DOH, Leeds, UK

Department of Health 1998b The new NHS – working together: securing a quality workforce for the NHS. DOH, London, UK

Department of Health 1999 Clinical governance: quality in the new NHS. DOH, Leeds UK

Department of Health 2000a The NHS plan: a plan for investment, a plan for reform. DOH, London, UK

Department of Health 2000b Meeting the challenge: a strategy for the allied health professions. DOH, London, UK

Department of Health 2000c Making The change: a strategy for the professions in healthcare science. DOH, London

Department of Health 2000d Making a difference: clinical supervision in primary care. DOH, Leeds, UK

Department of Health 2001 Working together – learning together. A framework for lifelong learning for the NHS. DOH, London, UK

Department of Health 2003a The Chief Health Professions Officer's ten key roles for allied health professionals. DOH, London, UK

Department of Health 2003b Level 5 dimension 20 – Management of people (31395). The NHS knowledge and skills framework (NHS KSF) and development review – working draft. DOH, London, UK, p 104. Online. Available: http://www.dh.gov.uk/assetRoot/04/07/37/ 48/04073748.pdf. Accessed 4/11/05

Department of Health 2004a NHS improvement plan 2004: putting people at the heart of public services. DOH, London, UK

Department of Health 2004b The NHS knowledge and skills framework (NHS KSF) and the development review process appendix 2: the NHS KSF dimensions, levels and indicators: core dimension 2: personal and people development for change, p 61. Online. Available: http://www.dh.gov.uk/assetRoot/04/09/08/ 61/04090861.pdf. Accessed 24/2/06

Department of Health 2006 Our health, our care, our say: a new direction for community services. DOH, London, UK

Department of Health (2006b) From values to action: The Chief Nursing Officer's review of mental health nursing. DOH, London, UK

Department of Health and Royal College of Nursing 2003 Freedom to practise: dispelling the myths. DOH & RCN, London, UK

Driscoll J J 2000 Practising clinical supervision: a reflective approach. Bailliere Tindall (in association with the RCN), Harcourt, London, UK

Driscoll J J, Cooper R 2005 Coaching for clinicians. Nursing Management 12(1):18–23

Edwards D, Cooper L, Burnard P et al 2005 Factors influencing the effectiveness of clinical supervision. Journal of Psychiatric and Mental Health Nursing 12(4):405–414

Ferguson K 2005 Professional supervision. In: Rose M, Best D (eds) Transforming practice through clinical education, professional supervision and mentoring. Elsevier Churchill Livingstone, Edinburgh, UK, p 293–307

Fowler J 1996 The organization of clinical supervision within the nursing profession: a review of the literature. Journal of Advanced Nursing 23:471–478

Freshwater D, Walsh L, Storey L 2001 Prison health care: developing leadership through clinical supervision. Nursing Management 8(8):10–13

Freshwater D, Walsh L, Storey L 2002 Prison health care: developing leadership through clinical supervision. Nursing Management 8(9):16–20

Gibson T M, Heartfield M 2005 Mentoring for nurses in general practice: an Australian study. Journal of Interprofessional Care 19(1):50–62

Gilmore A 2001 Clinical supervision in nursing and health visiting – a review of the literature. In: Cutcliffe J, Butterworth T, Proctor B (eds) Fundamental themes in clinical supervision. Routledge, London, p 125–140

Grant J, Kilminster S, Jolly B, Cottrell D 2003 Clinical supervision of SpRs: where does it happen, when does it happen and is it effective? Medical Education 37:140–148

Grauel T 2002 Professional oversight: the neglected histories of supervision. In: McMahon M, Patton W (eds) Supervision in the helping professions. Pearson Education, New South Wales, Australia, p 3–16

Greaves B 2004 Professional development of nursing: practice nursing. Work Based Learning in Primary Care 2:29–81

Grover M 2002 Supervision for allied health professionals. In: McMahon M, Patton W (eds) Supervision in the helping professions. Pearson Education, New South Wales, Australia, p 273–284

Gustafsson C, Fagerberg I 2004 Reflection, the way to professional development. Journal of Clinical Nursing 13:271–280

Hall D 1998 Supervision and the occupational therapy profession. Mental Health Occupational Therapy 3(1):10–13

Harder C et al 2005 Policy and procedures document – policy for clinical supervision. Darlington Primary Care NHS Trust, UK. Online. Available: http://www.darlingtonpct.nhs.uk/documents/uploaded/ClinicalSupervisionPolicy.doc

Hawkins P, Shohet R 2000 Supervision in the helping professions. 2nd edn. Open University, Buckingham, UK

Haynes R, Corey G, Moulton P 2003 Clinical supervision in the helping professions: a practical guide. Thomson Brooks-Cole, Pacific Grove, CA, USA

Higgins A, McCarthy M 2005 Psychiatric nursing students' experiences of having a mentor during their first practice placement: an Irish perspective. Nurse Education In Practice 5(4):218–224

HPC 2004 Continuing professional development: consultation paper. Health Professions Council, London

HPC 2005 Continuing professional development: key decisions. Health Professions Council, London

Hughes L, Pengelly P 1997 Staff supervision in a turbulent environment: managing process and task in front-line services. Jessica Kingsley, London

Hunter E, Blair S 1999 Staff supervision for occupational therapists. British Journal of Occupational Therapy 62(8):344–350

Hussain M 2004 Clinical supervision: implementing the framework from the College of Radiographers. Synergy (November):19–23

Hyrkas K 2005 Clinical supervision, burnout and job satisfaction among mental health and psychiatric nurses in Finland. Issues in Mental Health Nursing 26:531–556

Hyrkas K, Koivula M, Paunonen M 1999 Clinical supervision in nursing in the 1990s – current state of concepts, theory and research. Journal of Nursing Management 7:177–187

Johns C 2000 Becoming a reflective practitioner. Blackwell, Oxford

Kadushin A 1992 Supervision in social work. 3rd edn. Columbia University, New York, USA

Kadushin A, Harkness D 2002 Supervision in social work. 4th edn. Columbia University Press, New York, USA

Kilminster S M, Jolly B C 2000 Effective supervision in clinical practice settings: a literature review. Medical Education 34:827–840

Kirk S, Eaton J, Auty L 2000 Dieticians and supervision: should we be doing more? Journal of Human Nutrition and Dietetics 13:317–322

Kirkham M 1996 (ed) Supervision of midwives. Midwives Press, London

Lambert V, Glacken M 2005 Clinical education facilitators: a literature review. Journal of Clinical Nursing 14(6):664–673

Launer J 2003 A narrative based approach to primary care supervision. In: Burton J, Launer J (eds) Supervision and support in primary care. Radcliffe Medical, Oxford, UK, p 91–101

Maben J, Macleod-Clark J 1996 Preceptorship and support for staff: the good and the bad. Nursing Times 92(51):35–38

Malin N 2000 Evaluating clinical supervision in community homes and teams serving adults with learning disabilities. Journal of Advanced Nursing 31(3):548–557

Manley K, Hardy S, Titchen A et al 2005 Changing patients' worlds through nursing practice expertise: exploring nursing practice expertise through emancipatory action research and fourth generation evaluation. A Royal College of Nursing research report, 1998–2004. Royal College of Nursing Institute, London, UK

McDonald J 2002 Clinical supervision: a review of underlying concepts and developments. Australian and New Zealand Journal of Psychiatry 36:92–98

McMahon M, Patton W 2002 (eds) Supervision in the helping professions. Pearson Education, New South Wales, Australia

McSherry R, Pearce P 2002 Clinical governance: a guide to implementation for healthcare professionals. Blackwell, London

Mills J, Francis K, Bonner A, 2005 Mentoring, clinical supervision and preceptoring: clarifying the conceptual definitions for Australian rural nurses: a review of the literature. Rural Remote Health 5(3):410. Online. Available: http://rrh.deakin.edu.au/publishedarticles/article_print_410.pdf. Accessed 9/9/05

Morrison T 2003 Staff supervision in social care. Pavilion, Brighton, UK

Morton-Cooper A, Palmer A 2000 Mentoring in practice. In: Morton-Cooper A, Palmer A (eds) Mentoring, preceptorship and clinical supervision. 2nd edn. Blackwell Science, Oxford, UK, p 35–88

NHSCGST 2005 Clinical governance defined (NHS Clinical Governance Support Team). Online. Available: http://www.cgsupport.nhs.uk/About_CGST/Clinical_Governance_defined.asp. Accessed 29/11/05

NMAG 2004 Clinical supervision for mental health nurses in Northern Ireland: Best practice guidelines. Nursing and Midwifery Group, Department of Health, Social Services and Public Safety, Belfast, UK

Nursing & Midwifery Council 2005a Midwife's rules and standards. NMC, London

Nursing & Midwifery Council 2005b Supporting nurses and midwives through lifelong learning. NMC, London

O'Malley C, Cuncliffe E, Hunter S, Breeze J 2000 Preceptorship in practice. Nursing Standard 14(28):45–49

Page S, Wosket V 2002 Supervising the counsellor a cyclical model. 2nd edn. Brunner–Routledge, East Sussex, UK

Palsson M, Norberg A 1995 District nurses' stories of difficult care episodes narrated during systematic clinical supervision sessions. Scandinavian Journal of Caring Sciences 9:17–27

Paunonen M, Hyrkas K 2001 Clinical supervision in Finland – history, education, research and theory. In: Cutcliffe J, Butterworth T, Proctor B (eds) Fundamental themes in clinical supervision. Routledge, London, p 248–302

Power S 1999 Nursing supervision: a guide for clinical practice. Sage, London

Proctor B 1986 Supervision: a co-operative exercise in accountability. In: Marken M, Payne M (eds) Enabling and ensuring – supervision in practice. National Youth Bureau, Council for Education and Training in Youth and Community Work, Leicester, p 21–34

Rafferty M, Jenkins E, Parke S 2003 Developing a provisional standard for clinical supervision in nursing and health visiting: the methodological trail. Qualitative Health Research 13(10):1432–1452

RCSLT 1996 Communicating quality 2 – professional standards for speech and language therapists. Royal College of Speech and Language Therapists, London, UK

Rose M, Best D 2005 (eds) Transforming practice through clinical education, professional supervision and mentoring. Elsevier Churchill Livingstone, Edinburgh, UK

Royal College of Nursing 2005 Agenda for change. A guide to the new pay, terms and conditions in the NHS. RCN, London

Ryan S 2004 Vital practice – stories from the healing arts: the homeopathic and supervisory way. Sea Change, Portland, UK

Scaife J 2002 Supervision in the mental health professions. A practitioner's guide. Brunner-Routledge, Hove, UK

Scally G, Donaldson L J 1998 Clinical governance and the drive for quality improvement in the NHS in England. British Medical Journal 317:61–65

Schroffel A 1999 How does clinical supervision affect job satisfaction? The Clinical Supervisor 18(2):91–103

SCoR 2003a Clinical supervision: a position statement. Society and College of Radiographers, London, UK

SCoR 2003b Clinical supervision framework. Society and College of Radiographers, London, UK

Sellars J 2000 Supervise and reflect. Physiotherapy Frontline 6:20

Sellars J 2004 Learning from contemporary practice: an exploration of clinical supervision in physiotherapy. Learning in Health and Social Care 3(2):64–82

Severinsson E, Borgenhammar E 1997 Expert views on clinical supervision: a study based on interviews. Journal of Nursing Management 5(3):175–183

Severinsson E, Hallberg I 1996 Clinical supervisors' views of their leadership role in clinical supervision process within nursing care. Journal of Advanced Nursing 24:151–161

Skoberne M 2003 Supervision in midwifery practice. Midwives 6(2):66–69

Sloan G, Watson H 2002 Clinical supervision models for nursing: structure, research and limitations. Nursing Standard 17(4):41–46

Sood A, Driscoll J 2004 Clinical supervision in practice: a working model. Macmillan Voice (29): Spring (pull out-supplement), Macmillan Cancer Relief

Stevenson C 2005 Postmodernising clinical supervision in nursing. Issues in Mental Health Nursing 26:519–529

Stevenson C, Jackson B 2000 Egalitarian consultation meetings: an alternative to received wisdom about clinical supervision in psychiatric nursing practice. Journal of Psychiatric and Mental Health Nursing 7:491–504

Strong J, Kavanagh D, Wilson J et al 2003 Supervision practice for allied health professionals within a large mental health service: exploring the phenomenon. Clinical Supervisor 22(1):191–210

Sweeney G, Webley P, Treacher A 2001 Supervision in occupational therapy part 3: accommodating the supervisor and supervisee. British Journal of Occupational Therapy 64(9):426–431

Tate S, Richardson J, Leonard O, Paterson J 2003 Implementing clinical supervision for complementary therapy tutors: an evaluation. School of Integrated Health, University of Westminster, London, UK

Teasdale K, Brocklehurst N, Thorn N 2001 Clinical supervision and support for nurses: an evaluation study. Journal of Advanced Nursing 33:216–224

Thomas R 2005 Practice, legal principle and the supervisor. Practising Midwife 8(8):22–25

Titchen A 2003 Critical companionship Part 1. Nursing Standard 18(9):33–40

Titchen A, Binnie A 1995 The art of clinical supervision. Journal of Clinical Nursing 4:327–334

Todd G, Freshwater D 1999 Guided discovery and reflective practice: models for clinical supervision. British Journal of Nursing 8(20):1383–1390

Tudor K, Worrall M 2004 Freedom to practise person centred approaches to supervision. PCCS Books, Ross on Wye, UK, p 247–266

Weaver M 2001 Introducing clinical supervision. British Journal of Podiatry 4(4):134–143

Winstanley J 2000 Manchester clinical supervision scale. Nursing Standard 14(19):31–32

Winstanley J, White E 2003 Clinical supervision: models, measures and best practice. Nurse Researcher 10(4):7–38

Wood J 2003 Creative supervision. The Homeopath 91:28–30

Yegdich T 2002 Articulating the practice of clinical supervision in nursing. In: McMahon M, Patton W (eds) Supervision in the helping professions. Pearson Education, New South Wales, Australia, p 249–260

Yegdich T, Cushing A 1998 An historical perspective on clinical supervision in nursing. Australian and New Zealand Journal of Mental Health Nursing 7:3–24

2 Supported reflective learning: the essence of clinical supervision?

John Driscoll

INTRODUCTION

The previous chapter examined the increased legitimacy of clinical supervision and why its development and implementation is important in modern healthcare. This chapter continues that theme and, as in the previous edition, I persist with the idea that supported reflective learning is, in itself, the very essence of the clinical supervision encounter. However, in the spirit of reflection and acknowledging that the use of questions is central to the process of learning about reflection (Todd & Freshwater 1999), I pose some questions that I hope might be indicative of the sorts of questions you, the reader, might pose about reflection and reflective practice.

Throughout the chapter I use the term *reflection* as the process of going about reflection and *reflective practice* as it applies to the work of the health professional. While this is perhaps a simplistic way of looking at what is a complex concept, my purpose is to offer a starting point before addressing the question posed in the title of the chapter (Supported reflective learning: the essence of clinical supervision?). Using this as a platform, I begin to expose some of my own thoughts and understandings which you may, or may not, agree with and pose further questions about the relationship between reflective practice and clinical supervision. However, it is not my intention for this chapter to form a comprehensive literature review of reflective practice, as very readable analyses are available elsewhere (Bulman & Schutz 2004, Ghaye & Ghaye 2004, Johns 2002, Johns & Freshwater 2005, Rolfe et al 2001, Moon 2004, Tate & Sills 2004, Taylor 2005).

Writing the introduction to this chapter reminded me of how I used to initiate students into the subject of reflective practice at the beginning of a training programme by placing what I think is called a figure–ground illusion on the projector. As an example of the vagaries of the process of simple visual perception, it is a useful metaphor for the more complex vagaries of conceptual perception (e.g. 'seeing' reflective practice) (Figure 2.1).

There are at least three perceptual, or 'seeing', experiences evoked by the examination of Figure 2.1 and these experiences can also be evoked by the examination of the concept of reflective practice:

- Some of you might see it straight away.
- Some of you might see it if is pointed out to you.
- Some of you might still not see it despite it being pointed out to you.

(Just in case, I have placed what Figure 2.1 depicts after the On Reflection box at the end of the chapter!)

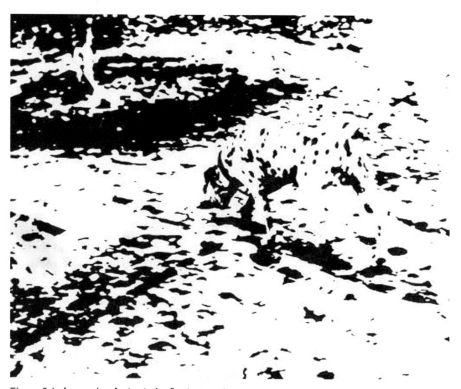

Figure 2.1 A metaphor for 'seeing' reflective practice

The point I am trying to make here, as I was with my students, is that some people cannot see the value of reflective practice straight away and sometimes even after they have had a chance to experience it they still fail to appreciate its value. As regards to this chapter the same is likely to apply and I encourage you to come to your own conclusions about whether reflection and reflective practice might be the essence of clinical supervision. In any event, I give you some of my personal signposts to help you make more sense of reflection and reflective practice and decide on whether utilizing clinical supervision in your practice will, or will not, assist you on your lifelong learning journey as a qualified health professional.

WHY THE NEED TO BE REFLECTIVE WHEN I ROUTINELY THINK ABOUT WHAT I DO IN MY CLINICAL PRACTICE?

Reflective practice is often seen as representing a choice for health professionals to be reflective or not to be reflective about their clinical practice, but as Bright (1995) suggests, in reality, such a dichotomy is false as everyone needs to engage in some form of self-reflection about their professional work. Although we will explore this in more detail later in the chapter, I suspect that many of you reading this might agree with the idea that as you think about your clinical practice as a matter of routine anyway there is no need to set aside specific 'reflective' time. This attitude presents a real challenge to health professionals as it hampers attempts to legitimize intentional reflection as an everyday activity in clinical practice. I tend to agree with Jarvis (1992), who points out that while no profession can claim to have reflective practice *per se*, what individuals within that profession have is an ability and a choice to practise reflectively. This does not mean that they will choose to reflect, only that the potential to do so exists within them.

So, although you may think you routinely reflect about your clinical practice, how often do you actually do so? I wonder how many of you when asked this question might sympathize with Smythe (2004), who questions whether there is even time to think, let alone be reflective, in busy work environments in which people are having to rush around from one demand to another in a world that expects an instant everything.

Reflection has a variety of definitions but which one you favour will depend on how relevant it is to your own situation. One of the best descriptions for me is given by Boyd and Fales (1983):

> … reflective learning is the process of internally examining and exploring an issue of concern, triggered by an experience, which creates and clarifies meaning in terms of self, and which results in a changed conceptual perspective …

So, according to this definition, reflecting on an experience is an intentional learning activity requiring an ability to analyse the self in relation to what has happened or is happening and make judgements regarding this.

However, what can pass for reflection might not be reflection; thinking about an experience or event is not always purposeful and does not necessarily lead to new ways of thinking or behaving.

Having recently moved house to a coastal area, I find I now can have greater distances to drive to places of work. Being new to the area, I am consciously aware of having to concentrate on the twists and turns of the comparatively narrow coastal roads. After I reach the main motorways I find that I am more relaxed because I feel I know where I am going and the roads are more familiar as well as wider. So, I go from being consciously aware of my driving, because the situation is unusual, to a more relaxed, almost automatic, mode of driving in the familiar surroundings of the motorways.

While I am no angel, it is interesting to note how many people I see on my travels engrossed in hand-held mobile telephone conversations, changing CDs, turning to others in the car or hunting in a glove compartment for something while driving. Perhaps I should pay more attention to what I am doing rather than observing others! (Unusually (thankfully), didn't I recently read about a woman applying her make up with both hands off the steering wheel? Wasn't she snapped by a road camera and didn't the image appear on the front pages of the tabloid papers?)

I suppose, like me, when those drivers started learning to drive they had to concentrate on what they were doing if they wanted to avoid collisions, never mind pass the test … but what of these people and myself now? … Has driving a car sometimes become so routine an activity that we don't have to think about it very much and can somehow switch on to 'auto-pilot'?

If I allow my driving behaviour to become an unthinking routine won't I increase the risk of having an accident (maybe lethal)? And here's the point, could the same complacency existing within the 'routine' behaviours of a health professional increase the risk of a 'professional accident'?

Of course reflection is not simply about managing the risk of healthcare; it is also an intentional method of learning which should lead to improvement in oneself and in one's practice.

In an increasingly patient-led UK health service (Department of Health 2005) health professionals are dealing with people who, because of their individual natures, require staff to be responsive and reflective instead of people who are simply carrying out what may seem like routine and repetitive tasks.

Although reflective practice is an opportunity to capture, examine and challenge some of the set patterns of working, such examination might lead to the realization that there is a need for change. This implies disruption and effort and it is much simpler to continue working in the same set ways — unless something unusual happens that forces some form of reflection. (For example, Jones (2004) cites a paramedic practice where there was a tendency to formally reflect on dramatic events but ignore the routine day-to-day things that they also dealt with — but I suggest that this is a feature of the reflective practice of many other health professionals new to the idea of practising reflection.)

In your own personal experience and based on what you have read so far, can you think of an example that illustrates when *you* (not somebody else) might have been on 'auto-pilot' or engaged in a routine activity in practice? What were you doing at the time?

What do you think some of the implications might be for being in this mode of practice for:
a) yourself as a health professional?
b) your colleagues?
c) the organization in which you work?
d) the person(s) you were treating or were caring for?

There will be moments, such as in emergency situations, where to physically stop and think in the midst of the action would be inappropriate and even life-threatening. But, in situations like these, formally replaying or having a debriefing session about the events at a respectable distance in time after the incident has occurred would be beneficial. Such reflections not only establish what went wrong but also affirm best practice.

While it is obviously unreasonable and physically impossible to continually reflect on everything that happens in practice, there are gains to be made in regularly stopping to think about everyday practice. Engaging in regular clinical supervision activities offers opportunities not only to have a self-dialogue about selected elements of practice but also to acquire new perspectives and/or mentally reframe familiar ways of working.

It also needs acknowledging at this stage of the chapter that reflective practice is not just confined to clinical supervision; reflective processes are likely to be just as valuable across the whole spectrum of the healthcare organization.

HOW DOES THE PROCESS OF REFLECTION RELATE TO LEARNING IN AND FOR PRACTICE?

For most healthcare professionals their first exposures to reflection and reflective practices are likely to occur in the formal education setting of their initial training, with an expectation that these practices will become features of their continuing professional development (Tate 2004:8). (For me it was while undergoing teacher training as part of the requirement to become a clinical teacher in neurosurgical nursing.)

At a macro level, the process of reflection and reflective practice could be seen to begin with education providers. United Kingdom universities and colleges of higher education are institutionally responsible for ensuring that appropriate standards are being achieved in the education of healthcare professionals. The Quality Assurance Agency (QAA), in partnership with the regulating bodies of healthcare professionals, periodically reviews teaching and learning activities and part of its remit is to ensure that provision is being made for reflection time so that the students will to be able to link theory and practice (Department of Health/National Midwives Council/NHS/Health Professions Council 2004).

Exposure to reflection and reflective practice is critical, not only for supporting the fledgling reflective practitioners during their education and training, but also in helping them view reflective activities as being just as important after their qualification and in their development as continual learners in practice. Beyond registration, reflective practices, including clinical supervision, are periodically audited under clinical governance (described in the previous chapter). Clearly, reflective practice as a strategic learning activity in the development of health professionals is a central plank supporting change and reform in healthcare organizations.

At a micro level, the process of reflection, beginning in an educational setting, is often grounded in experiential learning and learning from experience. Usher and Soloman (1999) make a distinction between the two:

- the former is an internal dialogue which constructs experiences in a particular way to give them meaning to the individual; that is, in a cyclical fashion knowledge and learning are derived from experiences and future experiences are given meaning from the gained new knowledge and learning;

- in the latter learning emerges from direct involvement in an everyday context, e.g. the 'live' supervision of a learner by someone more experienced and/or the observation by the learner of the practice of the experienced person (such as a mentor).

Although there are endless possibilities as a qualified health professional for 'live' supervision and learning from a new situation, here we concern ourselves with the stages in the process of reflection that have formed many reflective frameworks and have formed the basis of preparation for and offered structure to clinical supervision.

Moon (2004:115), after examining a number of experiential learning stages proposed by a number of theoretical authors, synthesized eight sequential stages in the process of reflection (Box 2.1) that a learner will necessarily travel through.

BOX 2.1	*The sequential stages of the process of reflection. Reproduced with permission from: Moon J (2004) A handbook of reflective & experiential learning: theory and practice. Routledge (Taylor & Francis)*

- the 'having of' the experience
- a recognition of the need to resolve something
- clarification of the issue
- reviewing and recollecting
- reviewing feelings/the emotional state
- processing of knowledge and ideas
- eventual resolution, possible transformation and action
- possible action

It will be noted that the reflective sequence requires learners to have the experience before returning to replay it in a classroom, either to themselves or in a clinical supervision situation.

One is struck by the need to be committed to this type of learning as a reflective practitioner. It incorporates being able to:

- describe what happened,
- detach oneself from the action, in order to look more objectively at the situation,
- process ideas and emotions.

The emphasis is towards learning and subsequent forward action, but it is likely that in order to learn, some 'unlearning' of favoured ways of working might need to take place.

If one's first exposures to reflection and reflective practice (in an educational setting) are to be of benefit and to inspire confidence in it as a positive method of learning, then one needs to be not only supported through the exposures but also challenged.

For many students, attempts at reflection are very likely to be assessable (removing the element of choice) and this may induce concern about the process. A key difference between reflecting as part of an assessed training programme and as a qualified health professional in clinical practice, I would suggest, is that in the former the learner has a limited choice as to whether to reflect or not — that potentially might limit learning or reduce it to a superficial exercise, which in turn could have implications for a clinical supervision situation after qualification.

In taking on the responsibilities for the continuance of reflection and reflective practice through clinical supervision as part of a continuing professional development activity, facilitators are preparing not only potential supervisees, but also supervisors.

It is also very likely, in relation to this, that facilitators themselves will be engaged in a peer process of reflection and support in order not only to experience the process first-hand but also to be in a better position to empathize with students, thus making these early exposures the hoped for, positive experiences.

It would seem that for reflective practice to make a difference, not only to individual health professionals but also to their clinical practice, it needs to be more than simply a process; it needs to include a commitment to action-ing that learning (reflexive action). In this respect, I agree with Atkins and Murphy (1993) that this might not necessarily involve acts that can be observed by others. The individual learner makes a commitment of some kind on the basis of what has been learned as action; no one can 'see' this decision to commit. Although it is the final stage of the reflective cycle, the commitment potentially begins the cycle again.

Clinical supervision (applied reflective practice) would seem to give qualified health professionals a legitimate opportunity to regularly stop and think in the midst of practice and, if there is a commitment to reflexive action in terms of improving that practice, then whole areas of healthcare could be transformed.

HOW MIGHT ENGAGING IN REFLECTION SPECIFICALLY SUPPORT THE WORK OF THE HEALTH PROFESSIONAL?

The late Donald Schon (1983, 1987) considered two kinds of knowledge that professionals use in practice:

- empirical or scientific knowledge (the basis for 'technical rationality'), and
- 'tacit knowledge'.

'Technical rationality' depends on the possession and utilization of logic and should be used by professionals in their practice. It is based on empirical and scientific knowledge (often developed in university or research environments). Within this technical–rational mode of thinking, it is anticipated that health professionals will apply 'theoretical' knowledge to solve their practical problems.

'Tacit knowledge', on the other hand, is 'taken for granted' knowledge. So, for professionals, technical rationality is perceived as the more appropriate way of thinking. However, while technical rationality is useful to explain practice 'as it should be', it often fails to address the complex nature of practice 'as it really is'.

Schon (1983:42) describes the complex nature of professional practice as the 'swampy lowland', where situations can become confusing 'messes incapable of technical solution'. In other words, while a practitioner from any discipline does require a sound theoretical and scientific basis from which to operate, this, in itself, does not always produce effective practice. It is within this quagmire of uncertainty and personal conflict that the more 'tacit' or intuitive knowledge of practice is realized, and this has been popularized as the 'theory–practice gap' debate (Ousey 2000, Rolfe 1996).

However, as Griffiths and Tann (1992) suggest, the distinction between theory and practice (or reflection and action) is not a gap or difference in knowledge, but a mismatch between the personally held beliefs of health professionals and publicly held theories; these mismatches are perceived as contradictions. Reflective practice, therefore, has been developed to help health professionals articulate their own beliefs and compare them to publically held theories and, thus, help them to make sense of the 'swampy lowland' of complex practice in which there appear to be more questions than straightforward answers.

Chris Johns (2005:2) in his definition of reflection offers hope to health professionals as he invites us to enter and fully embrace the conflict of contradictions contained in Schon's 'swampy lowlands of practice' rather than avoid it or simply use reflection as a bridge to cross the terrain:

> Reflection is being mindful of self, either within or after experience, as if a window through which the practitioner can view and focus self within the context of a particular experience, in order to confront, understand and move toward resolving contradiction between one's vision and actual practice. Through the conflict of contradiction, the commitment to realize one's vision, and understanding why things are as they are, the practitioner can gain new insights into self and be empowered to respond more congruently in future situations within a reflexive spiral towards developing practical wisdom and realizing one's vision as a lived reality. The practitioner may require guidance to overcome resistance or to be empowered to act on understanding.

Rather than avoiding conflict, reflection offers a focus as well as an opportunity to become more self-aware of the contradictions that exist between our personal visions for practice, or how we would like to practice, and the way we actually do. All health professionals reading this chapter, I suspect, will have their own personal knowledge and vision for practice and would, if they had the opportunity or the resources, want to work in that particular way. I would suggest that clinical supervision might be a way of not just testing your commitment to the process of reflection, but more importantly of begining to validate your own vision for practice.

In your own personal experience and based on what you have read so far, can you think of a significant experience that illustrates when *you* (not somebody else) got stuck in the swampy lowlands of clinical practice?

Write brief notes about a 'significant' experience that best describes and highlights for you some of the contradictions between how you are currently practising and what you would consider your own vision or more 'desirable' practice.

It is important to describe in your own words what is actually happening rather than trying to analyse what you thought was happening at the time ... we will continue with this later in the chapter.

The process of reflection has been linked to reducing the metaphorical gaps between theoretical and personal (or intuitive) knowledge and producing insights useful to an individual's practice. However, paradoxically, the notion of intentionally identifying or producing gaps in practice has been used to encourage reflective thinking. For instance, Teekman (2000) found that the theoretical setting of situational gaps (e.g. comparing and contrasting phenomena, recognizing patterns, categorizing perceptions or reframing situations about clinical practice) led to self-questioning to create further meaning and understandings.

Although there are many different types of reflection, two most commonly known are reflection-in-practice and reflection-on-practice (Schon 1991).

■ Reflection-in-practice occurs while events are unfolding in which the health professional observes what is happening in practice and intervenes and makes adjustments in a reasoned way in the midst of the action.
An example of this might be dealing with an emergency admission to a mental health unit where the person has presented in a disturbed state and is unwilling to stay in hospital. In this situation an experienced health professional simply deals with the situation, drawing on all their professional expertise (such as de-escalating techniques, using skilful interpersonal communication while at the same time observing for the safety of those in the immediate vicinity as well as the service user). All this time the health professional may not be aware of all the interventions used and why, provided the situation resolves itself.

■ At a point later they might revisit the situation and reflect on action.
Therefore reflection-on-practice occurs after the event and is retrospective.

Although two common types of reflection have been described, I would suggest that there is also a third type of reflection in that it is possible to reflect on a situation before an event happens in order to rehearse it. Here I might include discussing with a senior colleague a situation that has yet to be faced; an obvious example would be going for an interview for promotion.

While no one type of reflection is posited as any better than another, the most common type of reflection practised in both the educational setting and in practice is reflection-on-practice. The sequential stages (Box 2.1) would seem to offer a 'what' and 'how' for the process of reflection as well as 'why' engaging in reflection supports the work of the health professional. A summary of the key elements of the processes of reflection is contained in Box 2.2.

BOX 2.2	*A summary of the key elements of the processes of reflection*

- an intentional learning activity that can be done alone, or with others
- emphasizes the individual nature of a health professional's work in the context of the practice setting
- is often started off by a personal reaction to events
- often involves becoming engaged in a staged process of events
- is focused on examining specific elements of a health professional's work
- involves a commitment to action

WHAT ARE SOME OF THE CONDITIONS AND CONSEQUENCES OF BECOMING A REFLECTIVE LEARNER IN PRACTICE?

As previously stated, for the qualified healthcare professional working in practice, unlike the student in education, there is usually an element of choice — engaging in reflection or not.

In addition to choice, there obviously needs to be a commitment and a desire to ask questions about one's self and the way practice is carried out, particularly as a response to something that was puzzling or surprised you in practice.

- For some, the process of reflecting on their practice, despite it seeming to be a good idea, might not fit in easily with their own learning style and can manifest itself as passive resistance, e.g. being too busy, or not being able to find the time. (One of the ways in which you might make reflection easier to accept is to consider yourself working as a co-learner with others in a peer group. This is discussed in more detail in Chapter 8.)

- One of the common concerns about reflective practice and clinical supervision is about the possibility of publically exposing your thoughts and ideas and perhaps your vulnerabilities as a health professional. I again think of students who have had poor or 'unsafe' experiences in reflective practice:
  - the breaking of confidentiality, albeit unintentionally, or having felt humiliated by others in recounting their practice stories. Although such cases might be isolated incidents (in most cases a learning contract would have been drawn up), such experiences can tarnish getting going at all with reflective practice.

- Another concern, related to clinical supervision, is that specific elements of practice that have been reflected upon and documented might then constitute a form of organizational surveillance (Cotton 2001, Gilbert 2001) by making the health professional's clinical practice more visible.

In my experience of facilitating formalized reflective practice, as well as being in a reflective group myself, health professionals often gain by considering from the outset some of the benefits and challenges (Box 2.3) posed in becoming a reflective practitioner before then embarking on the reflective journey.

| BOX 2.3 | *Some of the benefits and challenges of becoming a reflective practitioner in practice. Reproduced with permission from: Johns C (2000) Becoming a reflective practitioner: a reflective and holistic approach to clinical nursing, practice development and clinical supervision. Blackwell Science* |

Benefits

- Enhances rather than competes with traditional forms of knowledge for professional practice.
- Can generate practice-based knowledge, as it is based on real practice.
- Values what professionals do and why they do it.
- Can help to make more sense of difficult and complex practice issues.
- Can be a supportive process by offering a formal opportunity to share practice issues with peers.
- Has improvements to service delivery at the centre of the reflective conversation.
- Focuses the practitioner on ways of becoming more effective in practice, as the reflective conversation is action based.
- Reminds qualified health professionals there is no end-point to learning about their everyday practice.
- Offers a practice-based learning activity that can contribute to meeting CPD needs.

Challenges

- Finding the time to engage in the process.
- Confronts the routineness of everyday practice.
- Can often mean being a lone voice.
- Being less satisfied with the way practice is carried out.
- Efforts towards improving practice rather than staying the same.
- Being labelled a troublemaker.
- Suggesting alternative ways of working.
- Often faced with making difficult choices.
- Poses more practice questions than answers.
- Finding that others may not have answers to practice concerns.
- Peer pressure to keep things as they are.
- Fear of rocking the boat in relation to future promotion or ambitions.

While it is perhaps transforming to learn from and challenge the way we act in practice, unlearning what routinely we have been doing requires practical support as well as courage. More than likely further support will be required to cope with the new challenges presented by re-viewing or pre-viewing clinical practice through a reflective lens.

Looking over what has been said in this chapter, what skills and attributes (that you have or need) will assist your development as a reflective practitioner?

There is a risk that, by producing lists of skills and attributes necessary to become reflective, readers can become, at best, bored with reading them or, at worst, develop an overwhelming sense that they will never be able to acquire the skills and attributes listed. Often the best thing is to simply have a go! As one of the forefathers of reflective practice, John Dewey (1929), succinctly stated:

> … we do not learn by doing … we learn by doing and then realising what came of what we did …

HOW MIGHT I INCORPORATE SOME OF THE IDEAS OF REFLECTIVE PRACTICE INTO A CLINICAL SUPERVISION SITUATION?

At this point of the chapter it is time to begin to examine how reflective practice might intersect with clinical supervision. While I accept that not all reflective practice is clinical supervision, I do think that all clinical supervision is to a greater or lesser extent reflective practice. Both have as their central intentions an action focus towards either improving or developing the individual health professional and, in turn, clinical practice within an environment that is both challenging and supporting. Of course, in clinical supervision, reflection is usually guided either by peers or, in an ideal situation, a supervisor who has been selected by the supervisee. By its nature, clinical supervision is usually entered into on a voluntary basis, indicating at least a potential for committing to the process of reflection. With this in mind I offer the following (Box 2.4) as being some of the ways in which the process of reflection can be incorporated into the clinical supervision encounter. You might decide that some items should be excluded or other items added.

BOX 2.4	*How the process of reflection can be incorporated into clinical supervision*
	■ Value yourself enough to take regular time out to reflect on practice.
	■ Find someone you feel comfortable with to support you in your practice.
	■ Identify pertinent practice stories to reflect upon.
	■ Use a reflective framework to get you started.
	■ Write as well as talk about what happens in everyday practice.
	■ Validate the value of regularly reflecting on your practice in clinical supervision.

Value yourself enough to take regular time out to reflect on practice

For most of you reading this, I suspect that at some point you have had an opportunity to engage in some form of reflection whether in an educational setting or simply as a response to events in practice that stopped you in your tracks and made you think. For some of you the idea of reflecting on practice in practice might be something you would choose to avoid! — but perhaps it might be worth considering two obvious questions:

- Why do you think it might be important to take regular time out away from practice to reconsider selected aspects of the work you have been doing?
- What might be the consequences for yourself of not doing so?

Going back to the swampy lowlands of practice described earlier in the chapter — you perceive apparent contradictions between theory and practice in what you are doing and would like to have some time to reflect about them, but your workload does not allow you to do so. Now ask the questions:

- Why do you think it might be important to take regular time out away from practice to reconsider the contradictions you have identified in your practice?
- What might be the consequences for yourself of not doing so?

Inevitably tensions arise, one of which will likely be between finding the time for reflective practice and 'getting the job done' (Eltringham et al 2000). Gilbert (2001) refers to this as working in a culture of 'selfless obligation' in which staff needs are a lower priority than service-user needs.

Another tension may arise between those who embrace change and those who prefer the *status quo*. Despite the potential of reflective practice to advance practice, its use is resisted by some. Mantzoukas and Jasper (2004) argue, powerfully, that the conscious raising of issues, by the act of reflecting on clinical practice, might bring about the need to re-order that practice and this is likely to present a threat to the equilibrium of ward life and encourage efforts to discredit reflection as a valid activity.

As you evaluate the concept of reflective practice, it would be interesting to get your response to an uncomfortable question posed by Hall and Davis (1999): is it ethical to practise without engaging in reflective practice?

A third type of reflection, 'reflection before practice', was described above — it is used as a rehearsal prior to an event happening; in this case preparing to begin regularly reflecting on your practice in practice:
- Based on what you have read in this chapter, what are the likely challenges facing you in getting started?
- What seem to be some of your priority issues that need tackling first?
- How might you begin to overcome these?
- What resources do you already have around you?
- What will be your first steps towards reducing these?

Find someone you feel comfortable with to support you in your practice

Despite the challenges presented in becoming a reflective practitioner in practice, I continually find it amazing how resourceful health professionals become if they value the process enough to actively seek it out.

It is essential to find a clinical supervisor to help guide your reflective activities. (Clinical supervision is often referred to as guided structured reflection and in some cases clinical supervision policy is also referred to as protected reflective practice (Greenwich TPCT 2005).)

Of course reflection can also be a solitary activity (I suspect many of you may relate to this as you are (or were) students on a course that requires the keeping of a reflective diary or portfolio of events) but even though individuals might be committed to learning from reflection and feel they can do so effectively on their own, there are benefits in working with a clinical supervisor. The clinical supervisor can provide:

- a focus for thoughts which might otherwise remain just a collection of confusing ideas;
- continuity in the form of some follow-up (as in the next meeting) as otherwise reflections might easily be forgotten;
- reminders that reflection is also about being response-able — there is commitment to action;
- new perspectives and understandings;
- opportunities for further reflection.

It is also worth mentioning here that where reflection is not specifically clinical supervision, the person supporting your reflections, perhaps a bit confusingly, might be a mentor, practice-based assessor, critical companion, preceptor or even your manager.

The elements of the clinical supervisory relationship are outlined in more detail in Chapter 4, but it is probably useful to offer a rationale for having someone, or a group, to guide and support your reflections on practice. Maddison (2004) suggests that without active support, students may become stuck within the reflective sequence (Box 2.1) and, therefore, there might be a significant loss of potential learning and opportunity for change. I also seem to remember reading the phrase *paralysis by analysis*, which aptly describes the situation in which there is plenty of thinking time in reflection but no forward movement! A key element of facilitating reflection is managing the balance between challenge and support.

In clinical supervision, where qualified health professionals disclose elements of clinical practice, too much challenge might be viewed as punitive, while too much support might be viewed as collusion. The whole point about facilitating reflection in clinical supervision is to aid practice improvement by helping supervisees to become more consciously aware of their practice. Often the situations being reflected upon are complex and in these cases facilitating reflection is brought about by actively listening and offering some feedback. This helps supervisees to reframe their thoughts or gain fresh perspectives that enable them to make more informed decisions about the situations they find themselves in.

Based on the work of Johns (2000:52), estimating the amount of guidance needed by the supervisee might also be a valuable reference point, for both the supervisor and supervisee, in evaluating the effectiveness of their efforts in the process of reflection (Box 2.5).

Identify pertinent practice stories to reflect upon

John Launer (2003:93) defines clinical supervision as:

> ... an opportunity for a professional to change a story about a working encounter by holding a conversation with another professional ...

BOX 2.5	*The need to guide reflection or a way of evaluating its effectiveness in clinical supervision? Based on: Johns C, Freshwater D (2005) Transforming nursing through reflective practice, 2nd edn. Blackwell Science*

- To expose contradiction and emphasize felt conflict.

- To expose and confront distorted self-understandings and self-limiting beliefs and to challenge the practitioner to look at situations from new perspectives.

- To unearth and understand the factors that have limited the ability to achieve one's vision and actual practice.

- To nurture a commitment that may have become numbed or blunted when working in 'unsympathetic' environments.

- To gain new insights and discover and explore new ways of responding within situations.

- To penetrate critical levels of reflection that may be outside the scope of the practitioner reflecting by herself.

- To support practitioners to become empowered to take appropriate action to resolve contradiction.

It might be interesting to note that John Launer is a UK general medical practitioner who promotes a narrative-based approach in primary care supervision with his colleagues. Of course the whole point of the story in clinical supervision is to invite change and it seems entirely suitable at this stage in the discussion for us to examine just what might be appropriate sorts of stories to reflect upon.

Using a story metaphor reminds me of how odd I think it is that on buying a new book some people like to go straight to the back page to see how the story ends. Perhaps it is just as odd for someone who comes into a clinical supervision session to reflect on an end-point already reached. Clinical supervisors who have already drawn conclusions before the stories have been told must be regarded with suspicion and supervisees who offer the same old familiar stories might be regarded as having not entirely prepared for the reflective sessions.

Either way, the ability of supervisees to recall a practice story, I would suggest, is an important supervisee skill and the active element of reflecting on practice with another person(s). The clinical supervisor pays attention to the story, being careful not to get too wrapped up in the content. The essence of any good story is in how it is told; the clinical supervisor then helps the supervisee to derive meaning and see the bigger issues that emerge from it.

Although many of the things I hear in clinical supervision are 'concerns', it is an interesting and sometimes a more challenging proposition to recount positive experiences. Clinical supervision can become a very negative experience and only serve to demoralize the supervisee if the focus is always on the downside of practice. It can be quite enlightening to recall something that you were pleased about. The focus can then change to become: 'in what way did you think this went well?' Exploring why something was successful can be a major source of learning as the supervisee begins to understand the answer to the question and tries to repeat the good practice.

An essential skill for the supervisee is in deciding which stories are important. This is not always straightforward, for a number of reasons:

- Not making a note of significant things that have happened in practice since the last clinical supervision session.
- Selectively or genuinely being unable to remember the situation as it happened some time ago.
- Using informal chats in practice as a substitute for clinical supervision.
- Not being used to reflecting on practice with others in any depth.
- Not realizing that a particular story is worth exploring.
- Being unwilling or anxious about exposing a particular aspect of clinical practice.

Many of the above can occur when you don't give yourself enough preparation time between clinical supervision sessions. Sometimes this preparation will need to be done away from the pressured work environment. Inadequate preparation will mean that a large proportion of clinical supervision time is spent mulling over past events, which can become tiresome and be difficult for either party to sustain for any length of time. Clinical supervision time might be better spent if you have already given some thought to different ways of developing issues that have emerged. In this way the process will inform and enhance your clinical practice.

Keeping a written record, rather than simply a mental note, of issues that crop up in your practice can be useful and need not be time-consuming. It could simply take the form of a collection of 'tabloid newspaper banner headlines' that you compile in practice to remind yourself of what went on.

This was how I initially organized my own reflections and the activity of thinking about what headline to match the story helped reinforce my memory of it, and helped me identify what was important about the practice incident to take with me to a clinical supervision session. This sort of written record with a banner headline and a write-up of what happened, with a space down the right-hand page to pull out key elements for further analysis, was my way of keeping a reflective journal.

For others, the act of writing rather than verbalizing what was going on might be very different. Many policies on clinical supervision now contain formats that include a reflective structure and possible content offering guidelines for those new to reflecting on practice but these can be contentious in respect to confidentiality and who has access to them. Very readable ideas about reflective writing and the keeping of journals can be found in Bolton (2005), Moon (2004), Jasper (2003), Rolfe et al (2001), and Taylor (2005). Reflective frameworks can also be a way of beginning to not just think but write reflectively and are discussed later.

Those of you new to reflection or clinical supervision, or who are unsure about what might be an appropriate issue to take to clinical supervision (which is very unlikely), could consider completing, at the end of your practice day, some of the sentences in Box 2.6.

Use a reflective framework to get you started

As Bulman (2004:165) wryly considers, although you might be filled with enthusiasm to begin the reflective journey, the dilemma of just where to start is

BOX 2.6	*Some ideas from your area of practice that might be worth reflecting upon in clinical supervision (for completion at the end of your practice day)*

- Something that went really well for me today was …
- I really felt professional today because …
- What really drove me mad today was …
- What I attempted to do today that I hadn't tried before was …
- A recurring pattern for me in my practice that I noticed today seems to be …
- Something that concerned me about what I did today was …
- What really puzzled me today was …
- If I had the chance to replay what I did today I would …
- I felt really stupid today about …

common. Many reflective frameworks are based on stages of the reflective process (Dennison & Kirk 1990, Driscoll 1994, Ghaye & Lillyman 1997, Gibbs 1988, Rolfe et al 2001), differing levels of reflection (Goodman 1984, Mezirow 1981), student experiences (Stephenson 2000) or forms of knowledge for practice (Johns 2005). While the use of reflective frameworks can be a useful way to get started, they might also limit more creative thinking by just adhering to a reflective recipe of key questions. Not surprisingly, as Burton (2000) notes, for more experienced practitioners following a structure for reflection can also be frustratingly prescriptive.

Despite this, in my view, and based on feedback from a number of health professionals new to the idea of formally reflecting on practice, questioning is a key that can open a door to altered perspectives for practice. For me, the keys to reflection and expanding oneself and practice in clinical supervision are:

- the use of questions,
- exploring answers to those questions in the context of clinical practice,
- witnessing new understandings, and
- working with the supervisee in a dynamic movement towards actively applying the learning that has (or is) taking place.

It is interesting to consider how the What? Model of Structured Reflection (Driscoll 1994) came to be through many lengthy discussions between myself and Ian Clift, a student colleague of mine undergoing teacher training. We were influenced by reflective teaching methods and a number of theorists in experiential learning who included Boud et al (1985), Dennison & Kirk (1990) and Kolb (1984). I recall one of our assignments was exploring the use of questioning and we were searching for key headings that represented the reflective cycle. We were stuck on the action element when Ian just said 'how about — now what'? From this, the What? Model of Structured Reflection evolved and, as they say, the rest is history.

What was fascinating and also rather embarrassing was almost seven years later to find that the What–So What–Now What question headings had previously been utilized by Terry Borton (1970) as part of an experiential curriculum development initiative in schools in the USA. (Of course, this was unbeknown to me some twenty-four years earlier!) From those early beginnings, these key headings have not only been used, but also, I am glad to say, continue to be developed by other authors in clinical supervision and reflective practice (Bond & Holland 1998, Rolfe et al 2001).

For my part, the intention was (and still is) to offer a pragmatic approach to reflection for those new to the concept; although I am now more influenced by action-based approaches to clinical supervision through my interest in coaching (this is outlined in another chapter).

It might be argued that in an effort to influence action or outcome the other components of the reflective process(es) (including description, emotional content and analyses) become overlooked or not seen as important. I hope that this is not the case in my supervisory work but I will need to bear this in mind, and urge those using the What? Model of Structured Reflection to do the same (Figures 2.2 and 2.3).

Johns's (2005) model of structured reflection (Box 2.7) seems to fit clinical practice because it has been developed and validated in practice. Attempts to fit clinical practice into other models of reflection may be less successful because structured reflection is such a complex and still not fully understood method of learning.

Perhaps you might wish to explore this for yourself in your own clinical supervision and experiment with the range of frameworks or even develop one for yourself.

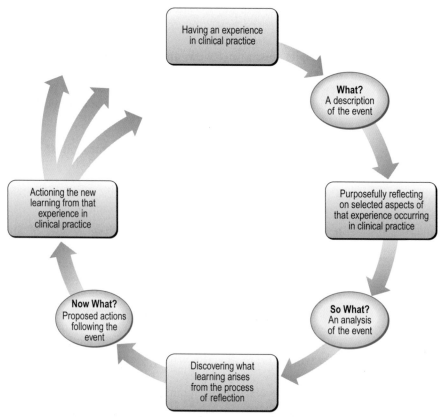

Figure 2.2 The What? Model of Structured Reflection and its relationship to an experiential learning cycle

1 **A *description* of the event**

What? trigger questions:

- is the purpose of returning to this situation?
- happened?
- did I see/do?
- was my reaction to it?
- did other people do who were involved in this?

2 **An *analysis* of the event**

So What? trigger questions:

- How did I feel at the time of the event?
- Were those feelings I had any different from those of other people who were also involved at the time?
- Are my feelings now, after the event, any different from what I experienced at the time?
- Do I still feel troubled, if so, in what way?
- What were the effects of what I did (or did not do)?
- What positive aspects now emerge for me from the event that happened in practice?
- What have I noticed about my behaviour in practice by taking a more measured look at it?
- What observations does any person helping me to reflect on my practice make of the way I acted at the time?

3 **Proposed *actions* following the event**

Now What? trigger questions:

- What are the implications for me and others in clinical practice based on what I have described and analysed?
- What difference does it make if I choose to do nothing?
- Where can I get more information to face a similar situation again?
- How could I modify my practice if a similar situation was to happen again?
- What help do I need to help me 'action' the results of my reflections?
- Which aspect should be tackled first?
- How will I notice that I am any different in clinical practice?
- What is the main learning that I take from reflecting on my practice in this way?

Figure 2.3 The What? Model of Structured Reflection and associated trigger questions

- You might now wish to complete the previous exercise that you began earlier in the chapter that centred on your journey through the 'swampy lowlands' of practice.
- Use either of the structured models contained in Figures 2.2 / 2.3 or Box 2.7 to reflect on your practice or as a preparation for a clinical supervision meeting.
- What was your choice of structured model and why?
- How helpful was it in helping you with your situation?
- What were the outcomes of your reflection-on-practice?

BOX 2.7	*Model for structured reflection (Johns 2005)*

Reflective cues	Way of knowing
Bring the mind home	Aesthetics
Focus on a description of an experience that seems significant in some way	Aesthetics
What particular issues seem significant enough to demand attention?	Aesthetics
How were others feeling and what made them feel that way?	Personal
How was I feeling and what made me feel that way?	Aesthetics
What was I trying to achieve and did I respond effectively?	Aesthetics
What were the consequences of my actions on the patient, others, myself?	Personal
What factors influenced the way I was feeling, thinking or responding?	Empirics
What knowledge informed or might have informed me?	Ethics
To what extent did I act for the best and in tune with my values?	Reflexivity
How does this situation connect with previous experiences?	Reflexivity
How might I respond more effectively given the situation again?	Reflexivity
Reflective cues	**Way of knowing**
What would be the consequences of alternative actions for the patient, others and myself?	Reflexivity
How do I *now* feel about this experience?	Reflexivity
Am I more able to support myself and others as a consequence?	Reflexivity
Am I more able to realize desirable practice monitored using appropriate frameworks such as framing perspectives, Carper's (1978) fundamental ways of knowing, other maps?	Reflexivity

PULLING IT ALL TOGETHER: IS SUPPORTED REFLECTIVE LEARNING THE ESSENCE OF CLINICAL SUPERVISION?

Clinical supervision would seem to give health professionals a legitimate opportunity to regularly stop and think in the midst of practice, with the intention of enhancing what already goes on in clinical practice. If actions occur by a supervisee as a result of guided reflection-on-practice with a clinical supervisor, or in a group situation, then clinical supervision through reflective practice may well be able to transform whole areas of clinical practice. While I readily accept that not all reflective practice is clinical supervision, I find it difficult to believe that it is possible to go about any form of clinical supervision without stimulating some sort of reflection or utilizing it as a reflective learning opportunity.

Fundamental elements of reflective clinical supervision are the development of skills and a demonstrable commitment by all parties to regularly work in this way. It is likely that the facilitator, guide or clinical supervisor not only would have first-hand experience of the process but also would have the skills, attributes and the confidence to guide the clinical supervision effectively. I would suspect that, in theory anyway, there already is a growing critical mass of individuals who might be more than happy to fulfil this role or are already doing so whether as supervisees or supervisors.

What if, as some authors suggest (Fowler & Chevannes 1998, Clouder & Sellars 2004), some health professionals do not wish to work in this way in clinical supervision or struggle with reflection, or have had less than positive experiences of working reflectively? And what of the newly qualified health professionals who want someone to 'really' supervise them, in the literal sense of the word, rather than engage in the hard work of reflection and self-development? What then?

Isn't clinical supervision also about feeling comfortable with the method and having a degree of choice? From an implementation perspective, what would be likely to happen if a method of reflection was imposed as clinical supervision? What if the thought of additional transformation, with so much change already happening in healthcare, is seen as likely to upset the equilibrium of healthcare delivery?

Transforming clinical practice through reflection is work in progress, not yet an everyday activity, but the number of health professionals learning to learn in this way is growing. While it might be liberating to learn from and alter the way we think and act in practice, unlearning what we have routinely been doing will require organizational as well as practical support. Therefore, it is important that all echelons of healthcare organizations have a collaborative vision for clinical practice and a belief that learning is a continuing process throughout a professional's life; as important at the top as at the lower end of of any healthcare organization.

The actions of senior staff in supporting practitioners who wish to be actively engaged in clinical supervision will be more important than the production of nicely worded policy documents. The notion of a lifelong learning culture in clinical practice, one in which there is freedom to learn and an openness to share first-hand experiences through reflection and clinical supervision as well as do the work, I would suggest, is the longer-term goal for any modern healthcare organization and legitimized by clinical governance. I wonder what might be the implications for you, the reader, in your own practice if such a goal were to be achieved?

On reflection ... chapter summary

- Supported reflective practice remains the essence of clinical supervision although not all clinical supervision is reflective practice.
- All health professionals have a reflective potential but this does not necessarily mean they will engage in reflective practice(s), only that a potential exists.
- Facilitating reflection in clinical supervision is to aid professional and practice improvement by helping the supervisee become more consciously aware of their practice.
- Rather than avoiding conflict, reflective practice offers a focus as well as an opportunity to become more self-aware of the contradictions that exist between how we envision practice and the way we actually carry out practice.
- For reflective clinical supervision to be realized in practice it will require organizational support to do so.

Figure 2.1 is a Dalmatian dog!

REFERENCES

Atkins S, Murphy C 1993 Reflection: a review of the literature. Journal of Advanced Nursing 18(8):1188–1192

Bolton G 2005 Reflective practice writing and professional development. 2nd edn. Sage, London, UK

Bond M, Holland S 1998 Skills of clinical supervision for nurses. Open University, Milton Keynes, UK

Borton T 1970 Reach, touch and teach. Hutchinson, London, UK

Boud D, Keogh R, Walker D 1985 Reflection: turning experience into learning. Kogan Page, London, UK

Boyd E, Fales A 1983 Reflecting learning: key to learning from experience. Journal of Humanistic Psychology 23(2):99–117

Bright B 1995 What is reflective practice? Curriculum 6(12):69–81

Bulman C 2004 Help to get you started – reflecting on your experiences. In: Bulman C, Schutz S (eds) Reflective practice in nursing. 3rd edn. Blackwell, Oxford, UK

Bulman C, Schutz S (eds) 2004 Reflective practice in nursing. 3rd edn. Blackwell, Oxford, UK

Burton S 2000 A critical essay on professional development in dietetics through a process of reflection and clinical supervision. Journal of Human Nutrition and Dietetics 5:317–322

Carper B 1978 Fundamental patterns of knowing in nursing. Advances in Nursing Science 1(1):13–23

Clouder L, Sellars J 2004 Reflective practice and clinical supervision: an interprofessional perspective. Journal of Advanced Nursing 46(3):262–269

Cotton A H 2001 Private thoughts in public spheres: issues in reflection and reflective practices in nursing. Journal of Advanced Nursing 36:512–519

Dennison B, Kirk R 1990 Do, review, learn apply: a simple guide to experiential learning. Blackwell Education, London, UK

Dewey J 1929 Experience and nature. Grave, New York

Department of Health 2005 Creating a patient-led NHS: delivering the NHS improvement plan. DOH, London, UK

Department of Health/National Midwives Council/NHS/Health Professions Council 2004 The partnership quality assurance framework for healthcare education in England: ongoing quality monitoring and enhancement (OQME) of healthcare education in England (standard 7.9 aspect 7: learning & teaching). DOH, NCM, NHS, HPC, London, UK

Driscoll J 1994 Reflective practice for practise – a framework of structured reflection for clinical areas. Senior Nurse 14(1):47–50

Eltringham D, Gill-Cripps P, Lawless M 2000 Challenging values in clinical supervision through reflective conversations. In: Ghaye T, Lillyman S (eds) Effective clinical supervision: the role of reflection. Quay Books, Wiltshire, UK, p 19–44

Fowler J, Chevannes M 1998 Evaluating the efficacy of reflective practice within the context of clinical supervision. Journal of Advanced Nursing 27:379–382

Ghaye A, Ghaye K 2004 Teaching and learning through critical reflective practice. David Fulton, London, UK

Ghaye T, Lillyman S 1997 Learning journals and critical incidents: reflective practice for health professionals. Quay, Wiltshire, UK

Gibbs G 1988 Learning by doing: a guide to teaching and learning methods. Oxford, UK

Gilbert T 2001 Reflective practice and clinical supervision: meticulous rituals of the confessional. Journal of Advanced Nursing 36:199–205

Goodman J 1984 Reflection and teacher education: a case study and theoretical analysis. Interchange 15(3):9–26

Greenwich TPCT 2005 Clinical supervision (protected reflective practice) policy. Greenwich Teaching Primary Care Trust, London, UK. Online. Available at: www.greenwichpct.nhs.uk/publications/file .aspx?int_version_id=1030. Accessed 31/10/05

Griffiths M, Tann S 1992 Using reflective practice to link personal and public theories. Journal of Education for Teaching 18(1):69–84

Hall M, Davis M 1999 Reflections on radiography. Radiography 5:165–172

Jarvis P 1992 Reflective practice and nursing. Nurse Education Today 12:174–181

Jasper M 2003 Beginning reflective practice – foundations in nursing & healthcare. Nelson Thornes, Cheltenham, UK

Johns C 2005 Expanding the gates of perception. In: Johns C, Freshwater D (eds) Transforming nursing through reflective practice. 2nd edn. Blackwell Science, Oxford, UK, p 1–12

Johns C 2002 Guided reflection: advancing practice. Blackwell Science, Oxford, UK

Johns C 2000 Being and becoming a reflective practitioner. In: Johns C (ed) Becoming a reflective practitioner: a reflective and holistic approach to clinical nursing, practice development and clinical supervision. Blackwell Science, Oxford, UK, p 34–67

Johns C, Freshwater D (eds) 2005 Transforming nursing through reflective practice. 2nd edn. Blackwell Science, Oxford, UK

Jones I 2004 Using reflective practice in the paramedic curriculum. In: Tate S, Sills M (eds) The development of critical reflection in the health professions. Learning and Teaching Support Network (LTSN) Higher Education Academy Health Sciences &

Practice, London, UK. Online. Available at: www.health.ltsn.ac.uk/publications/occasio nalpaper/occasionalpaper04.pdf, p 39–46. Accessed 02/02/06

Kolb D A 1984 Experiential learning: experience as the source of learning and development. Prentice-Hall, New Jersey, USA

Launer J 2003 A narrative based approach to primary care supervision. In: Burton J, Launer J (eds) Supervision and support in primary care. Radcliffe Medical, Oxford, UK, p 91–101

Maddison C 2004 Supporting practitioners in the process of reflection. In: Bulman C, Schutz S (eds) Reflective practice in nursing. 3rd edn. Blackwell, Oxford, UK, p 73–91

Mantzoukas S, Jasper M 2004 Reflective practice and daily ward reality: a covert power game. Journal of Clinical Nursing 13:925–933

Mezirow J 1981 A critical theory of adult learning and education. Adult Education 31(1):3–24 (an imprint of Taylor Francis Books, London UK)

Moon J 2004 A handbook of reflective & experiential learning: theory & practice. Routledge (Taylor & Francis), Abingdon, UK

Ousey K 2000 Bridging the theory–practice gap? The role of the lecturer/practitioner in supporting pre-registration students gaining clinical experience in an orthopaedic unit. Journal of Orthopaedic Nursing 4:115–120

Rolfe G 1996 Closing the theory–practice gap. Butterworth-Heinemann, Oxford, UK

Rolfe G, Freshwater D, Jasper M (eds) 2001 Critical reflection for nursing and the helping professions. Palgrave, Basingstoke, UK

Schon D 1991 The reflective practitioner – how professionals think in action. Avebury, Aldershot, UK

Schon D 1987 Educating the reflective practitioner. Jossey Bass, San Francisco, CA, USA

Schon D 1983 The reflective practitioner. Basic Books, Harper-Collins San Francisco, CA, USA

Smythe E 2004 Thinking. Nurse Education Today 24:326–332

Stephenson S 2000 Students' perspectives on reflective practice. In: Burns S, Bulman C (eds) Reflective practice in nursing: the growth of the professional practitioner. Blackwell Science, London, UK, p 124–136

Tate S 2004 Using critical reflection as a teaching tool. In: Tate S, Sills M (eds) The development of critical reflection in the health professions. Learning and Teaching

Support Network (LTSN) Higher Education Academy Health Sciences & Practice, London, UK, p 8–17. Online. Available at: www.health.ltsn.ac.uk/publications/occasionalpaper/occasionalpaper04.pdf. Accessed 30/11/05

Tate S, Sills M 2004 (eds) The development of critical reflection in the health professions. Learning and Teaching Support Network (LTSN) Higher Education Academy Health Sciences & Practice, London, UK. Online. Available at: www.health.ltsn.ac.uk/publications/occasionalpaper/occasionalpaper04.pdf. Accessed 30/11/05

Taylor B 2005 Reflective practice: a guide for nurses and midwives. 2nd edn. Open University, Buckingham, UK

Teekman B 2000 Exploring reflective thinking in nursing practice. Journal of Advanced Nursing 31(5):1125–1135

Todd G, Freshwater D 1999 Reflective practice and guided discovery: clinical supervision. British Journal of Nursing 8(20):1383–1389

Usher R, Soloman N 1999 Experiential learning and the shaping of subjectivity in the workplace. Studies in the Education of Adults 31(2):155–163

2 GETTING GOING WITH CLINICAL SUPERVISION IN PRACTICE

3 Boundaries and responsibilities in clinical supervision

Stephen Power

INTRODUCTION

Anyone who has ever asked a good friend to listen while they divulge a pressing problem will have some idea of the benefits of being a clinical supervisee. Hopefully, their friend will have been attentive, concerned and, possibly, even constructively helpful. The person with the problem may have been given 'food-for-thought' and now see their difficulty from a changed, more positive perspective. They may be encouraged, enlightened and enriched with new insights!

We would, surely, all want a friend like that! A friend who knew how to listen without missing the important bits; how to offer advice only when it was asked for — and then only if it was considered totally necessary; how to keep the conversation on the right track, without veering off on irrelevant tangents; how to avoid dominating the discussion with their own issues; how to bring the conversation to a controlled close; how to prevent being interrupted by the mobile phone playing The Entertainer; and especially, a friend who didn't have to leave right in the middle of the most important part of what you had to say, because the children were due to be collected from school.

Our friends want to do their very best for us. Often, though, there are limits to what they can do, paradoxically, because there are often no limits on the way that they do it. Friends rarely say: 'I've got exactly 20 minutes to talk to you' or 'I'll turn off the phone' or 'let's go for a coffee, but only if there is no one else in the café' or 'come and see me every other Tuesday at 4 o'clock'. The free-and-easy approach that our friends may adopt could very well result in us getting exactly the help we want, or it might leave us feeling pleased with our friend for offering — and trying — to do something for us, but also somewhat frustrated and with a sense that our business is still 'unfinished'.

Meeting with your clinical supervisor is not the same as talking to a friend. While it could well be a friendly encounter, there are good reasons why clinical supervisors should aim to do the very things that friends would never dream of doing. They should limit what they can do, and when they can do it. If clinical supervisors want to be more than a friend to their supervisees, they need to do what friends will never do to us — impose limits on their interactions with supervisees. However, in clinical supervision, limits are important and, when used carefully, will serve to enhance the quality of the experience.

A useful adage for clinical supervision might therefore be:

Less is more and more-or-less is not good enough!

Just like a house, any clinical supervision arrangement is likely to collapse very quickly without a strong foundation to support it. Without a carefully considered infrastructure – which includes agreed roles, responsibilities, boundaries and a contract that confirms all of those factors — clinical supervision runs the risk of becoming a friendly chat that can leave the supervisee feeling un-heard, un-helped and even more confused and frustrated than ever before. It is essential that the clinical supervisor gives a great deal of attention to designing and building the infrastructure to his work with a new supervisee, before the supervision work begins in earnest.

- How many of you reading this are currently engaged in clinical supervision without having negotiated any agreement or set boundaries beforehand with your clinical supervisor?
- What might be the consequences of you continuing in clinical supervision without having negotiated any agreement or set boundaries beforehand with your clinical supervisor?

Boundaries bring an element of consistency to the clinical supervision process. In my view, this leads to another very important reason for applying boundaries to a clinical supervision arrangement, and it is this:

Consistency generates trust. Trust generates rapport. Rapport generates progress.

Unless the clinical supervision arrangements are maintained consistently, it will be very difficult for both parties, and for the supervisee in particular, to begin to feel safe and 'trusting' within the professional relationship. As with most relationships, personal or professional, a degree of trust is required in order to allow rapport to develop. It is the rapport — a connection or bond — between the participants that allows for the development of a sense of security and safety, and an open and honest exchange of views and ideas. It is only when both parties in the supervisory arrangement feel that the situation is safe enough for them to be as open, honest and as frank as possible that they will really begin to work at their best, together.

For any clinical supervision arrangement to be sustained in practice, boundaries and responsibilities will need to be discussed and agreed before the supervision begins in earnest, and outlined in a way that is meaningful and easily understandable. The main elements of any supervisory agreement will then form the basis of what is called The Clinical Supervision Contract. Most clinical supervision contracts are written down and signed, although some supervisors may prefer to use a verbal contract.

This rest of this chapter will contain a discussion of the basic components of a clinical supervision infrastructure, including the necessary boundaries that might be set in place and the roles and responsibilities of both the supervisee and the clinical supervisor. I will finish by outlining some of the ways in which clinical supervisors might prepare and use a clinical supervision contract.

THE BOUNDARIES OF CLINICAL SUPERVISION

Boundaries are everywhere in everyday life. We are aware of them every time we fly to another country for a holiday or when our child's ball flies across the fence into next door's garden. In sport, the boundary lines mark out the area into which the play must be confined. Cross those lines and the game stops. It is worth considering that even the most fervent soccer fan will accept that a goal does not count if a player in his team was 'offside' at the time. In clinical supervision boundaries are used to indicate where we are (metaphorically), how and where the work will be carried out and what is considered to be 'fair play' and what is 'offside'.

Heru et al (2004) state that the boundaries of the supervisory relationship are important concerns and that the maintenance of good boundaries between trainees and supervisors is crucial to the integrity of the supervisory relationship. I have described, below, four main boundaries that can be used to build an infrastructure for clinical supervision. I refer to these as the boundaries of: Relationship; Content; Time; Space and Confidentiality. Each of these boundaries has, within it, a sub-set of parameters that are used by the clinical supervisor and supervisee to determine the limits within which they can operate.

The first meeting

During their first meeting, before any proper supervision work has begun, both parties need to establish enough information to enable them to be sure that they wish to at least begin working together in clinical supervision. My suggestion would be to set such a meeting up with the sole intention of gathering this information, and establishing the other boundaries to be discussed below, perhaps calling it a 'pre-contractual meeting' or similar name to imply that supervision will only start once the basic ground rules have been discussed and agreed.

For each boundary, below, I have raised a series of questions that can be used to set these pre-determined limits, and I have, in some cases, made suggestions as to how they might be applied. Final decisions on what are applicable boundaries should be made in agreement by individual supervisors and supervisees, as individual circumstances may have a bearing on the decisions made. It should be remembered, however, that clinical supervision is a professional relationship with the ultimate aim of enhancing the supervisee's clinical work. If that principle is borne in mind it will also soon become apparent that, in this model at least, the roles and responsibilities of both the clinical supervisor and supervisee are closely intertwined with the various boundaries. By answering the questions below, both parties will not only be setting the limits of their input, but also be defining why they are participating, what they can offer and what they cannot offer.

The boundary of relationship (1)

Before clinical supervisees can feel comfortable enough to work with their supervisors, they need to have some sense of who they are speaking to. And, before going any further, I feel that it is important to state the obvious — supervisees are allowed to ask questions. Unfortunately, while it may be a perfectly reasonable statement, it is not uncommon for both participants to assume that only the clinical supervisor should be asking questions. In many supervision arrangements it is often an implicit assumption that the clinical supervisor is automatically in a 'one-up position' in relation to the supervisee — perhaps due to a more senior professional standing — and is the only one allowed to ask questions about professional experience and expertise.

I totally disagree with this premise; I would go further and state that not only are supervisees allowed to ask pertinent questions of the clinical supervisor, but also that they should be encouraged to use those questions as the basis for a decision on whether they wish to continue working with that particular clinical supervisor, in the future.

What sorts of important information might the supervisee need to obtain from their clinical supervisor before agreeing the supervisory relationship?
- Who is the clinical supervisor?
- What is the clinical supervisor's experience of clinical supervision for healthcare workers?
- What is the clinical supervisor's specialist area(s) of clinical experience and expertise?
- What does the clinical supervisor expect from the supervisee in relation to the clinical supervision?

I have listed some typical questions that the supervisee might ask, together with an outline of the information that can be gleaned from asking them, in Box 3.1.

BOX 3.1	*Information for the supervisee to gather: Who is the clinical supervisor?*

- What is your name (what would you like me to call you?)
- Where do you work and what do you do there?
- How long have you been in your present post and where else have you worked recently that might have given you experience relevant to your supervision of me?
- What do you think that clinical supervision is about?
- How much experience do you have of supervising people in my clinical field?
- Do you prefer any particular model or style of clinical supervision?
- Do you have any specific training in clinical supervision?
- What would be the *minimum* length of time that you could reasonably commit to supervising me?

The answers given to such questions will be very useful in allowing the supervisee to gain a greater understanding of the clinical supervisor. The clinical supervisor's experience and knowledge (both clinical and supervisory) and their particular way of working might be apparent not only in the answers themselves, but in the way they are given. Similarly, the observant supervisee may be able to glean a sense of whether the clinical supervisor is someone who is seriously interested in the process of clinical supervision and committed to supervising them.

Before the end of the first meeting, the clinical supervisor should also have gathered enough information to feel reasonably certain that they understand at least something of the following:

- Who is the supervisee?
- What does the supervisee expect to gain from being supervised?
- Why does the supervisee want supervision now?

If they are to answer these key questions fully, the clinical supervisor will need to seek answers to a range of equally pertinent questions. I have listed some typical questions that the clinical supervisor might ask in Box 3.2.

BOX 3.2	*Information for the clinical supervisor to gather: Who is the clinical supervisee?*

- What is your name (what would you like me to call you)?
- Where do you work and what do you do there?
- What other clinical experience do you have?
- Have you been supervised previously?
- Why have you chosen me for your clinical supervisor?

The answers that the supervisee gives to the questions will be very helpful in allowing the clinical supervisor to understand a number of things about the supervisee, including their current level of clinical experience and — consequently — whether they are appropriately qualified and experienced enough to supervise them. The clinical supervisor may also find it helpful — and possibly enlightening — to have a sense of what the supervisee expects to get out of the process of clinical supervision, both specifically and generally, and why the supervisee has chosen them. Answers to this question might range from an unrealistic, idealized view of the clinical supervisor, at one extreme, to an apathetic, 'stuck-for-choice' response, at the other extreme. The clinical supervisor is likely to be encouraged by a more balanced and well-considered answer than either of those.

The boundary of content

The boundary of content, to use a sporting analogy, is used to determine when the supervisory 'ball' is in — and out — of 'play'. Within this boundary are contained all the issues that will be considered 'fair game' for the supervisory process. Once the clinical supervisor and supervisee discuss and agree what can be brought to supervision, they will know, by omission, those areas that cannot be considered. And it should be remembered that this boundary applies to both parties.

It would be very tempting to see clinical supervision as your own personal space, in which you can talk about whatever you like: holidays; relationship problems; changing physical appearance; application for another healthcare post, all spring to mind as potential 'grist for the mill'.

The short answer is: any topic that has a direct connection to my being a healthcare professional. Some topics may be more obvious than others and present themselves more readily to the clinical supervisor. Talking about a television drama to my clinical supervisor might seem like a pointless and time-wasting exercise, but what if it featured a character that reminded me of a client that I am working with, and had triggered off several new ideas about my work with that person? It might suddenly become relevant and a new source of information to assist the supervisory process.

Jones (2001) feels that clinical supervision involves establishing professional relationships that are concerned with safe and effective (clinical) practice. He states that it is important that clinical supervisors and supervisees are able to work together constructively and he goes on to say that clinical supervisors and supervisees should consider their roles and responsibilities outside of supervision and how these might influence the supervision relationship.

Hawkins and Shohet (1989:55) have described four main elements involved in clinical supervision (*see* Box 3.3). Although most clients never attend supervision with the supervisee, these four elements will always be present, either in a real and tangible way, or in some other way — usually through talking, thinking and feeling something about them. That said, I have, in the past, been involved in 'live' client-present clinical supervision where the client has listened to the clinical supervisor and supervisee discuss the clinical assessment. The clinical supervisor has a responsibility for guiding the supervisee toward thinking about the client and helping to maintain a connection between the supervisee, the client, the working environment and the clinical situation.

BOX 3.3	*The key elements in clinical supervision*
	■ The clinical supervisor
	■ The supervisee
	■ The client (or the work, generally, being undertaken)
	■ A work context

An essential responsibility, within the boundary of content, is for the clinical supervisor to decide if they are up to the task of offering the supervisee what they are expecting to get from supervision. The clinical supervisor needs to consider if they have the appropriate clinical experience and professional background to match with the supervisee's own background, professional orientation and level of experience. They also need to consider if their personal style of supervision — the models they use, and their theoretical orientation — fits the needs of that particular supervisee. Relevant questions that the clinical supervisor might ask the supervisee are outlined in Box 3.4. Some psychological frameworks are discussed in Chapter 5.

It is not enough for supervisors to assume that they will be able to offer their own particular brand of supervision to every supervisee they meet.

BOX 3.4	*Information for the clinical supervisor: What does the supervisee want?*

- What does the supervisee want from clinical supervision?
- Why is the supervisee asking for clinical supervision at this particular point in their career?
- How does the supervisee see me?
- What does the supervisee expect to get from me?
- Are they reasonable expectations?
- Am I in a position to offer what the supervisee wants?

The boundary of relationship (2)

In an ideal healthcare world, the clinical supervisor and supervisee would not meet outside of the carefully pre-arranged time of the supervision session itself. They would not debate the best course of action for a new client at a case conference, overhear each other's conversations in the dining room or even bump into each other at the local pub. In an ideal world, both parties would not know each other outside the confines of the clinical supervision room, and the supervision process itself would occur in a pure form, free from the intrusive clutter of the real world and unencumbered by embarrassment, pride and concerns about being seen to be 'good enough'.

But, things are different in the real world. Not only do clinical supervisors and supervisees often have professional (and possibly personal) contact with each other outside supervision, one may even be working closely with the other — and even have managerial responsibility for them. If supervision is to be practised in a way that allows both parties —and in this case, especially the supervisee — to feel relaxed and safe about the process, I suggest that close attention should be given to applying 'the boundary of relationship'.

One way of thinking about this boundary is to see it as a guide to what each person can expect from the other, and also what they cannot expect. A good starting point for deciding this is to refer back to the boundary of content, above. By applying the boundary of content, it is impossible for the clinical supervisor and supervisee to discuss anything that is not, in some way, related to the supervisee's clinical practice. So, with this parameter in place, it becomes easier for the clinical supervisor to decide what can (and cannot) be offered to the supervisee.

The clinical supervisor's responsibility here is to ensure that only clinical supervision is offered in the clinical supervision session. Idle chit chat is not appropriate; neither is gossip, managerial supervision or therapy.

If the supervisee wants to talk about going on holiday, for example, the clinical supervisor might ask questions like: How long will you be away? What affect will this have on your clients? Will you need to ask someone to cover your caseload? What do you feel about leaving your work behind you? All of those questions are designed to assist the supervisee in thinking about the specific relationship between the holiday and the clinical work. However, the clinical supervisor should be discouraged from asking: Did you get a good deal on the flight? Are you going with your partner? Have you been there before? Do you like Italian food? Those questions have nothing to do with the clinical work of the supervisee and take the conversation down a particularly 'chatty' and an un-supervisory road. While supervision might be carried out in a friendly manner, the clinical supervisor has a responsibility to ensure that the supervision process does not become simply a 'chat' between 'friends'. Supervisors should be constantly alert to when the conversation is drifting away from the central focus, of the supervisee's work, and do all they can to bring it back.

If the supervisee begins to talk about a personal relationship difficulty or other domestic problems — perhaps issues about bringing up their children — the clinical supervisor's responsibility is, once again, to make the connection between the material presented and its bearing on the supervisee's clinical work. If it has no bearing on the clinical work, the supervisee should be, gently, encouraged to find another forum for working on those issues. There may be other decisions to make regarding issues that are obviously very important to the supervisee, but which have no direct relation to their clinical work. As tempting as it might be, especially for practitioners working within the mental health field, supervisors should not allow themselves to be drawn into becoming the supervisee's therapist, counsellor or 'agony aunt'.

However, there may be a pressing issue for the supervisee that is hard to ignore because it keeps reoccurring, but which does not have a 'work context', and therefore clearly sits outside this boundary. In that case, the clinical supervisor has a responsibility to bring attention to it and, as carefully as possible, suggest that the supervisee might consider seeking professional counselling or some other appropriate form of help with the difficulty.

In the previous edition of this book, a number of other erroneous models of supervision, arising out of the clinical supervisor's lack of understanding of — and preparation for — the role, were described (Driscoll 2000:67, Box 5.3). These include:

- The Road Works Model, where the clinical supervisor tells the supervisee which direction to take in their practice;
- The Firefighter Model, which has the clinical supervisor attempting to dampen down the metaphorical 'smouldering fires' that occasionally flare up in practice; and
- The Great Pretender Model, in which the clinical supervisor avoids confrontational issues with the supervisee, and gives the impression that everything in the supervisory garden is rosy — all of the time.

These practices, and other equally unhelpful ones outlined by Driscoll, are not conducive to the facilitation of successful clinical supervision and should be avoided at all costs.

In some healthcare settings, the organizational situation may demand that the clinical supervisor is also managerially responsible for the supervisee. As a clinical supervision *purist* I am not in favour of this arrangement, and would strongly discourage it, as it has the potential to cause confusion and consternation for both parties. I am aware of more than one supervisee who has become disenchanted with the process, very quickly, due to the clinical supervisor's insistence on talking about duty rosters, overtime, holiday cover and even raising professional conduct and disciplinary issues in what should be a space for thinking solely about the supervisee's clinical work.

The confusion between clinical supervision and managerial supervision is, in my view, probably the single most important reason why clinical supervision fails to become fully implemented within some healthcare organizations and a key reason, frequently cited by supervisees, for personal dissatisfaction with the process. Some healthcare line managers who provide clinical supervision for their teams are — or at least, *believe* they are — able to 'switch' from one role to the other — and back again — with consummate ease. I know of one line manager who talks to supervisees about 'taking my manager's hat off and opening my clinical supervisor's ears'. Such an approach is to be commended, but it does have potential pitfalls:

- Even when the clinical supervisor can genuinely resist the urge to speak like the supervisee's line manager, they may still think like a line manager — and this will not be lost on the supervisee.

- Many supervisees will be extremely uncomfortable about bringing anything to supervision that might cause their clinical supervisor/manager to see them in 'a bad light'.

- The supervisee has to think to the future and their career development. There are promotions, references and annual performance reviews to consider.

- The anxiety surrounding giving a good impression — or, at least, not giving a bad one — to the 'boss' can be so stultifying as to render supervisees virtually speechless when faced with their clinical supervisor/manager.

For me, the notion of a solid structure — or framework — within which to practise clinical supervision is of paramount importance. Without such a structure, supervision would be chaotic and confused, to say the least. When we consider the key elements that go to make up this structure, the boundary of relationship has to be seen as one of the most vital. An understanding of it ensures that both parties are clear about their individual roles and responsibilities within the supervisory process, and — as importantly — what they are not expected to do. In Box 3.5, I have outlined what the clinical supervisor might do — and not do — with the supervisee to help reinforce the boundary of relationship.

BOX 3.5	*Some ways to maintain the boundary of relationship*

Clinical supervisors should encourage supervisees to *only* discuss:

- Anything that is directly related, or connected to, the supervisee's clinical work with clients, patients or colleagues or the clinical work in general.

The clinical supervision process should not contain elements of:

- A friendly chat
- Gossip

During a clinical supervision session it is not appropriate for supervisors to act out the role(s) of:

- Therapist
- Counsellor
- Agony aunt
- Line manager

In the next section, I will look at another fundamental boundary of clinical supervision, that of time, and how it might be used most effectively.

The boundary of time

Many sporting events start — and stop — when the referee blows his whistle and last precisely as long as is stipulated by the rules. The venue is always fixed well in advance and there are a pre-determined number of matches in a 'season' or cup competition. While it might be disadvantageous to see clinical supervision as a competitive 'sport', some of the same principles apply to arranging a meeting between clinical supervisor and supervisee.

Applying the boundary of time to a clinical supervision contract allows both the supervisee and supervisee to make, in agreement between themselves, important decisions about the venue, frequency and duration for the supervision work. Without this important 'boundary', any supervision arrangement runs the risk of becoming disorganized, disjointed and very disagreeable.

In order to apply the boundary of time appropriately, I suggest that the clinical supervisor and the supervisee discuss and then answer the questions below, in a way that is — as far as possible — appropriate to, and manageable by, both of them. It would be unwise to propose that only the clinical supervisor's needs are to be taken into consideration when setting the boundary of time. If the supervisee feels pressured into agreeing to an arrangement that is unsuitable for them, the supervision arrangement is likely to break down quickly and, possibly, irreparably. Some key questions to consider regarding the boundary of time can be summarized as:

■ When (and where) will each clinical supervision session take place?

■ How often and for how long?

■ How many sessions?

■ How long will each session last?

When (and where) will each clinical supervision session take place?

The clinical supervisor and supervisee should try, as far as possible, to arrange a regular time to meet. If the time for each session can be agreed in advance, even for only a few sessions at a time, it will serve the purpose of allowing the supervisee to feel more supported and secure in their supervision.

Similarly, the place for each session should be agreed in advance and adhered to as far as possible, for as long as possible. If either party wants to change the time of the meeting, it should be done as far in advance as possible.

How often and for how long?

The questions of how frequently clinical supervision session should occur, and how long each session should last, are crucial to the overall success of the experience. The answers will often depend on a number of factors including: organizational constraints; the amount of clinical work each supervisee is bringing;

and whether the supervisee will be seen alone or in a group. Generally, consideration of the following points may be useful when planning the length and frequency of supervision sessions with a supervisee:

- The amount and intensity of the supervisee's clinical work.
- The availability of the clinical supervisor.
- The constraints and existing policies of the organization.

- How will you find the time for regular and formalized clinical supervision in busy practice?
- What might be the consequences of:
  a) doing so, and
  b) not doing so?

How many sessions?

There are few standard 'bench-marks' in terms of clinical supervision session frequency. One model that exists, from the practice of psychoanalysis, is to halve the number of hours spent seeing clients (or patients) and to spend that time in supervision. This usually requires a weekly attendance at clinical supervision. For many practitioners, however, especially those in NHS settings, this is a totally impractical suggestion.

As a starting point, I would suggest holding clinical supervision sessions every four weeks. Some healthcare workers may prefer a shorter frequency (perhaps meeting fortnightly) and some, either by necessity or through choice, may desire even longer gaps between sessions.

Winstanley and White (2003) conducted a validation study of the Manchester Clinical Supervision Scale and recommended that supervision sessions should be monthly or bi-monthly in frequency.

How long will each session last?

As with the frequency of sessions, the length of each clinical supervision session must be agreed at the first meeting between clinical supervisor and supervisee and before the work 'proper' begins. Once these times have been agreed, it is the responsibility of both parties to ensure that it is applied to each and every subsequent clinical supervision session.

A popular time, per individual clinical supervision session for healthcare workers, seems to be forty-five minutes. Some healthcare workers trained or training in psychotherapy prefer the so-called psychoanalytic hour, which lasts, somewhat confusingly, for fifty minutes. It is so-called because some therapists with large caseloads, and a requirement to schedule several patients 'back-to-back' in any one day, find it beneficial to leave ten minutes or so between appointments for 'thinking time' and for recording the session. Winstanley and White (2003) suggest that clinical supervision sessions should last for one hour, and that they could be extended by a further thirty minutes for community practitioners. Sloan (2005) recommends that perhaps the nursing profession needs to consider establishing a minimum amount of supervision for its practitioners. This would appear to be a suggestion that would be appropriate for all healthcare professionals to consider. Sloan also recommends negotiating a protocol for cancellations and a procedure for contacting the clinical supervisor in an emergency situation.

Both the clinical supervisor and supervisee should try not to let clinical supervision sessions over-run and do what they can to avoid starting late. An important responsibility for the clinical supervisor is to ensure that the session is gently, but firmly, ended as close to the agreed time as possible.

A useful strategy for good time-keeping in clinical supervision sessions is to keep a clock or watch in sight during the session, perhaps by taking off a wristwatch and putting it on the desk. The clinical supervisor may wish to announce the amount of time left, as the end of the session approaches, by saying something like, 'we have got ten minutes left, is there anything else you would like say that you haven't already mentioned?' This can have the effect of helping the supervisee to consolidate their thoughts, which will assist in bringing the session to an orderly and satisfying conclusion.

The boundary of space

When thinking about the boundary of time, it is important to consider the associated concept of the boundary of space. I use this term to refer to the environment within which the time will be spent. This is about not only the physical space (the room itself, and its location) but also the quality of that space, and the potential of it to promote a high standard of clinical supervision work. It is a responsibility of the supervisor to consider the location of the room itself, and its suitability to the task of supervision.

The questions below are raised with the intention of assisting clinical supervisors in their selection of a suitable venue. Issues concerning the location of the room, whose room it is, its size and furniture and the potential for disturbance when in the room can be crucial to the perceived quality of the supervision process and should not be considered as insignificant to the planning process. Some key questions to consider regarding the boundary of space can be summarized as:

- Where will clinical supervision happen?
- Finding a room.
- Can you eliminate or reduce the prospect of interruption?

Where will clinical supervision happen?

The question of where the supervision will take place can be addressed from two perspectives. Firstly, is the room on the clinical supervisor's 'patch' or will the clinical supervisor travel to meet the supervisee? Answering this question automatically determines who has responsibility for 'managing' the room; ensuring that it is available at the required times and suitably prepared for each session.

Secondly, the clinical supervisor needs to know whether or not there is enough available space in their office or usual place of work. Also, is where the clinical supervisor regularly works too busy or too noisy to consider making it the venue for supervision? If they usually work in an open-plan office environment, for example, can they find a big enough room to use on a regular basis?

Finding a room

Can you have the same room at the same time on a regular basis or will you need to book different ones? Having to book rooms for each separate session can lead to confusion and disruption of the sessions, if it is not properly managed. Supervisees need to feel that they are being attended to by the clinical supervisor and that their needs are paramount, at least for the time set aside for *their* clinical supervision.

If it is necessary to book different rooms for each supervision session, try to do it for the whole year, or another considerable 'block' of time, and not from one session to another. Giving this block of dates to your supervisee, in order that she knows where she will be several weeks in advance, can go a long way to establishing a sense of containment and assurance in the supervisee.

Can you eliminate or reduce the prospect of interruption?

It is important that you do everything possible to ensure that you will not be inappropriately disturbed during the supervision session. Interruptions can come from so many different places, often all at once, that it will be difficult to prepare for all of them, but it is important that, as a clinical supervisor, you consider that for the period of the supervision session it is your number-one priority other, perhaps, than for certain very specific and predetermined events for which you are prepared to be contacted. If there are issues that you consider important enough to be contacted about during supervision sessions, make sure you have a clear idea what these are and tell whoever is likely to contact you well in advance.

The boundary of confidentiality

Another important responsibility that both the clinical supervisor and the supervisee will need to acknowledge is one that I call the boundary of confidentiality. This is potentially the most confusing and misunderstood of all the boundaries of clinical supervision. Although the interest in clinical supervision appears to be flourishing, there has been a concern among some theorists that the potential minefield of legal, accountability and ethical issues may be making the road from passive interest to practice one that is too difficult for many healthcare professionals (Cutcliffe et al 1999).

Supervisees will, no doubt, be concerned that their privacy and rights to confidentiality will be protected during the supervision process. For many supervisees, the supervisory relationship is unlikely to be successful if trust cannot be established early and maintained throughout the duration of the process. However, there is more than just the supervisees' rights to confidentiality to be considered.

There are at least three people involved in the process of clinical supervision: the clinical supervisor; the supervisee; and the client. In some cases, the word 'client' might represent a single person, a couple, a family, a small group of people, or even a large caseload of clients. Everyone that a particular clinical supervision session refers or relates to is entitled to expect that their rights to confidentiality are recognized and, where appropriate, are upheld. For this reason, many supervisees are encouraged to seek the permission of their client(s) before bringing their work to a clinical supervisor. Some models of clinical supervision (and some clinical supervision contracts) require explicit, often written, permission from clients that their material can be presented to clinical supervisors before the process can begin. Some clinical supervisors, who receive clinical supervision themselves, may also make a similar request of their supervisees. Naturally enough, this stringent requirement can make the whole process so much like a metaphorical minefield that many practitioners don't even consider it as an option at all. Similarly, the clinical supervisor has a right to expect that any material of a professional or personal nature disclosed to the supervisee may also be treated with respect and held in confidence.

It is also necessary for both the clinical supervisor and the supervisee to understand that it may be appropriate, under certain, previously agreed circumstances, for the confidentiality rule to be broken. At the contracting stage (see below), and before formal clinical supervision begins, a frank discussion should take place about the use of confidentiality within supervision and its inherent limitations. An important responsibility here is for both the clinical supervisor and supervisee to agree on the circumstances under which confidentiality must be broken and how this should be done. Any proposed breach of confidentiality deemed necessary by the supervisor should be discussed in full with the supervisee. What I am referring to, specifically, is the question:

To what extent will confidentiality be applied and maintained during the clinical supervision process?

If clinical supervisors say to supervisees 'everything you tell me will be held in the strictest confidence', they are likely to be demonstrating a serious lack of understanding of the nature of confidentiality as it applies to their employing organization and possibly also giving the supervisee a false sense of indemnity from professional misconduct. It follows, therefore, that while all supervisees might consider that they are entitled to have any issues raised during clinical supervision protected from being disclosed to anyone outside the process, it is important to consider under what circumstances the clinical supervisor might feel compelled to discuss the supervisee's work (or behaviour) with a third party. Local healthcare organization policies will, in the first instance, probably be the best guide to making decisions about how far the boundary of confidentiality can extend within any particular clinical supervision arrangement.

As a starting point, clinical supervisors might agree with their supervisees that the boundary of confidentiality could be broken when a matter raised is deemed (by either one of them) to be illegal, in breach of either party's professional code of conduct or infringes on the employing organization's disciplinary and/or complaints policies and procedures. In addition, the clinical supervisor and supervisee may wish to agree at the outset of the clinical supervision sessions that the clinical supervisor will advise the supervisee to report the misconduct to the relevant authority himself. It could be agreed, and even included in the supervision contract, that the clinical supervisor will report the matter if she is satisfied that the supervisee has failed do so themselves, at the earliest opportunity.

The recording of information in a professional healthcare context is another sensitive and often contentious issue that is an integral part of the boundary of confidentiality. The possible legal and ethical implications of making and keeping notes about clinical supervision sessions also need to be given much careful consideration.

Important questions for the clinical supervisor and supervisee to consider include:

- Will the clinical supervision session records be made available to anyone other than the clinical supervisor and supervisee?
- Are there circumstances under which it might be appropriate to show the written record of the clinical supervision sessions to a third party?
- Who else might be entitled to demand to see a written record of the clinical supervision sessions?

Once again, these considerations may appear so off-putting as to scupper the clinical supervision process before it begins. But, if a reliable evaluation system of the process of clinical supervision is to be established, then some sort of record will need be kept. Dimond (1998a) has suggested that the employer resourcing the provision of the clinical supervision should have the right to receive: 'The minimum necessary information for effective monitoring to take place.' Dimond further cautions nurses considering setting up clinical supervision systems that: 'if disciplinary proceedings were to be brought against either the clinical supervisor or supervisee then the complete supervision record might have to be made accessible to the employer if it is relevant to an issue arising in the proceedings' (Dimond 1998a). She adds that if the clinical supervision sessions take place during working hours — which is the most desirable option — then the ownership of the records themselves will reside with the employer. Dimond also states that courts may be in the position of subpoenaing clinical supervision notes, other than when information is exempt from disclosure on grounds of legal professional privilege.

My suggestion for record keeping in clinical supervision (Power 1999) is that the supervisor should keep a very brief record of each supervision session, perhaps detailing the following information:

- The date of the clinical supervision session.
- The time it began.
- The time it ended.
- The names of those attending the clinical supervision session.
- A brief, general, note of the issues raised and discussed.
- The agreed date of the next clinical supervision session.

This record would not contain specific personal information on patients or any other information that could identify individuals. It is rarely necessary, in my experience, for supervisees to use more than a person's first name, whether that person was a patient, colleague or other associate. I have also managed to retain enough information about the details of the sessions by using code words or letters of the alphabet, in any records that I have kept.

Some clinical supervisors advise their supervisees to keep a diary of reflective practice to which they can refer during clinical supervision sessions. In addition, supervisees may wish to keep reflective diaries specifically referring to the supervision sessions, as an adjunct to, and a reminder of, the clinical supervision itself. Again, Dimond (1998b) warns that such notes may, in certain circumstances, be required to be made available to the courts. It would be unfortunate though, in my view, if concerns of a legal nature prevented clinical supervisors or supervisees from keeping reasonable records of clinical supervision sessions, as many will value the benefit of a written reminder or *aide-mémoire*. If supervisors and supervisees take care over what, how and where they record the process of their clinical supervision sessions, it will lead to increased input, and output, and informed evaluation of the whole process.

Similarly, when the boundary of confidentiality is recognized as a tool to enhance the safety and security of the clinical supervision process, rapport is likely to increase and the supervisory process will be enhanced. Once it is fully explored, understood, defined and agreed at the beginning of the clinical supervision process, the boundary of confidentiality will no longer be seen as a threat or a reason to abandon clinical supervision. On the contrary, an awareness of the need for this boundary and an acceptance of it should lead to a more open supervisory relationship in which both participants treat each other as responsible adults.

THE CLINICAL SUPERVISION CONTRACT

Once they have been agreed to by both parties in the clinical supervision process, the ground-rules that I have discussed above will form the basis of the Clinical Supervision Contract. The intention of the contract is to help bind both parties to the arrangements and agreements that have made during the preliminary clinical supervision meeting. The contract is a two-way agreement, which should contain a strong element of joint ownership within it. If the contract is not made with the whole-hearted and equal input of both the clinical supervisor and supervisee any agreements reached are likely to be quickly breached. The process of drawing up the contract will help make the process more defined and explicit for both the clinical supervisor and clinical supervisee, and drawing it up together will strengthen the ownership of it. Wilkin (1998) states that the supervision contract: 'basically … encourages a reciprocal relationship-orientated approach, whilst outlining the boundaries and individual responsibilities of both clinical supervisor and supervisee'.

While the clinical supervision contract can be made verbally, many clinical supervisors and their supervisors prefer to have written versions of the contract which is signed by both parties at the first session and copies of which are held by both parties as an *aide-mémoire*. Taking the time to do this can lead to a consolidation of the professional relationship between the clinical supervisor and the supervisee. It also helps to avoid any later confusion around just what was agreed. However, Sloan (2005) states that the drawing up and keeping of documentation is an aspect of clinical supervision that can instil a great deal of anxiety in the supervisee. He feels that this concern often relates to who will keep (and, presumably, view) the documentation, what information will be recorded and for what purpose it will be used.

A typical method of drawing up the clinical supervision contract would be for the clinical supervisor and supervisee to talk about the boundaries in turn and then agree on the extent and limitations of each of them. It might then be a

simple matter of stating in the contract that both parties have agreed to 'Work within the boundary of relationship as previously discussed', and so on for each boundary. Other clinical supervisors might prefer to clearly state each element of each boundary on a separate sheet of paper, which both parties would sign. This method, while very thorough, might be considered too time-consuming and unnecessarily fastidious for many participants.

Whatever method of making the contract is chosen, it is vital that both the clinical supervisor and supervisee have discussed, fully understood and agreed on all of the important components. Howard (1997) suggested a twelve-item clinical supervision agreement checklist. This includes the following points:

- Purpose
- Professional disclosure statement
- Practical issues
- Goals
- Methods and evaluation
- Accountability and responsibility
- Confidentiality and documentation
- Dual relationships
- Problem resolution
- Statement of agreement

In Box 3.6, I have offered a template for a clinical supervision contract, which is reasonably typical of those used by a number of healthcare organizations. This contract includes many of the essential components necessary and can be used, at the very least, as a starting point for developing more specific ones. Healthcare professionals should consider what fundamental information they would need to include in contracts for use in their own organizations, and alter the template accordingly. Ultimately this decision needs be made by those healthcare professions who are leading the development of clinical supervision in the relevant organizations, with very specific reference to the organization and its personnel.

BOX 3.6	*A template for contracting in clinical supervision*

ANYTOWN HEALTHCARE N.H.S. TRUST
CLINICAL SUPERVISION CONTRACT (page 1)

THIS CONTRACT WILL COMPLEMENT THE TRUST POLICY
AND GUIDELINES ON CLINICAL SUPERVISION

CLINICAL SUPERVISEE: John Smith

DESIGNATION: Occupational Therapist

CLINICAL SUPERVISOR: Jane Brown

DESIGNATION: Clinical supervisor

BOX 3.6	*(Cont'd)*

VENUE: Interview Room, Health Centre.

TIME/FREQUENCY: Every two weeks, for one hour.

REVIEW OF SUPERVISION:

Every six months, between clinical supervisor and supervisee. New contract to be signed after the review.

CLINICAL SUPERVISION CONTRACT (page 2)

JOINT RESPONSIBILITIES:

1. To honour the contract.

2. To maintain the boundaries of Relationship; Content; Time; Space and Confidentiality, as discussed and agreed to in the preliminary supervision meeting.

CLINICAL SUPERVISOR'S RESPONSIBILITIES:

1. To provide supervision as per policy and guidelines.

2. To record each client discussed in supervision on a recording sheet after each session.

3. To record the time and date of each supervision session on a recording sheet after the session.

SUPERVISEE'S RESPONSIBILITIES:

1. To accept supervision as per policy and guidelines.

2. To prepare material to be discussed, in advance of the supervision session.

3. To pre-select suitable clients for presentation at the supervision session.

NOTE:

a) Supervision sessions will only be cancelled due to sickness, or if making the session becomes impossible for either party.

b) If the need for supervision arises outside contracted sessions, a clinical supervisor will accommodate the supervisee as soon as possible for an extra session.

NB: The boundaries of confidentiality within supervision are anything that is illegal, that breaks the individual's professional code of conduct or infringes the Anytown Healthcare N.H.S. Trust Disciplinary Policies.

SIGNED:

Clinical Supervisee..................................... Date..

Clinical Supervisor..................................... Date..

On reflection ... chapter summary

- Limits are important in clinical supervision, and serve to enhance the quality of the supervisory experience.
- The structure of the clinical supervision process is defined by its various boundaries and the limitations of those boundaries.
- The boundaries of clinical supervision include the boundaries of relationship; content; time; space; and confidentiality.
- A clinical supervision contract can make the process more explicit.
- Drawing up a contract together can help consolidate the ownership of it.

REFERENCES

Cutcliffe J, Epling R M, Cassedy P et al 1999 Ethical dilemmas in clinical supervision 1: need for guidelines. British Journal of Nursing 7(15):920–923

Dimond B 1998a Legal aspects of clinical supervision 1: employer vs employee. British Journal of Nursing 7(7):393–395

Dimond B 1998b Legal aspects of clinical supervision 2: professional accountability. British Journal of Nursing 7(8):487–489

Driscoll J 2000 Practising clinical supervision: a reflective approach. Baillière Tindall, London

Hawkins P, Shohet R 1989 Supervision in the helping professions. Open University, Milton Keynes

Heru A M, Strong D R, Price M, Recupero P R 2004 Boundaries in psychotherapy supervision. American Journal of Psychotherapy 58(1):76–89

Howard F M 1997 Supervision. In: Love H, Whittaker W (eds) Practice issues for clinical and applied psychologists in New Zealand. The New Zealand Psychological Society, Wellington, p 340–358

Jones A 2001 The influence of professional roles on clinical supervision. Nursing Standard 15(33):42–45

Power S 1999 Nursing supervision: a guide for clinical practice. Sage, London

Sloan G 2005 Clinical supervision: beginning the supervisory relationship. British Journal of Nursing 14(17): 918–923

Wilkin P 1998 Clinical supervision: the Rochdale support and development model. Rochdale Healthcare NHS Trust, Rochdale

Winstanley J, White E 2003 Clinical supervision: models, measures and best practice. Nurse Researcher 10(4):7–38

4 Essential elements for a successful supervisory partnership to flourish

Daniel Nicholls

INTRODUCTION

In this chapter I hope to show that the supervisory relationship involves a creative act. Often creativity involves knowing how to put things together, like taking pieces of a puzzle and putting them together into a meaningful whole. When you read this chapter, for example, you put together various ideas (from both you and me) and come to a creative understanding — something slightly (or very) different from what we previously understood. John Driscoll thought the ideas in this chapter could be put together like a jigsaw puzzle, so he gave me an idea for a couple of diagrams to represent the initial chaos of ideas and the (almost) finished product that you'll find represented at the end of the chapter. Thanks John! You'll see that some of the sub-sections of the chapter are longer than others. The reason for this is that not all of my thinking is evenly distributed (my internal *sentences* are not of equal length or share the same spaces — thus you'll see repeated themes popping up all over the place). This chapter should never be the final word on any matter but the start of a discussion that continually develops … like clinical supervision. You will thus notice that the grammatical person shifts between 'I', 'we', 'one' and 'you'. We are all the same in many ways, yet I am different from you as one can only be different from another (Figure 4.1).

The creative act in clinical supervision is about how we ask questions of others and ourselves. The creative act first requires a change or transformation. With this book, for example, we see a transformation of the First Edition into the Second. John Driscoll has already described the conditions for ideal supervisory relationships in the First Edition. One of the principal themes that emerged there was 'active noticing' (Driscoll 2002:89), a pervading essential skill for both

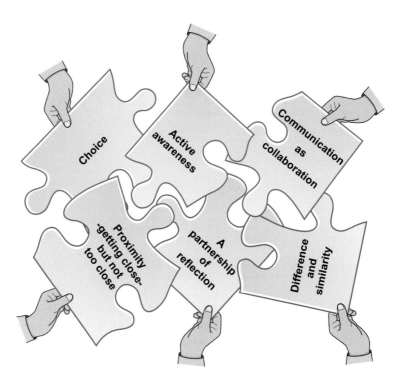

Figure 4.1 The puzzle of the supervisory relationship

supervisor and supervisee. Here, I shall build a little on this theme and describe ways in which this activity can 'become real' in an act of creation. In order to create, however, we need to have an idea of where we are located in our thinking. That requires that we ask ourselves questions about things we often take for granted. A good place to start is to look at the words we use and how we use them.

In order to start this process let's take a look here at just two words in the title of this chapter: the verb *to flourish*. What does *to flourish* mean? 'Thrive, prosper, be successful.' I think an earlier meaning can also be resurrected: up to the mid-eighteenth century it was: 'Display vigour, *in*, *with*' (Brown 1993). For clinical supervision is not about passivity. It is an active engagement, requiring energy and vigour.

Pesut and Herman (1999:11), in discussing clinical reasoning, draw a useful distinction between action and reflection. For them, reflection follows action. For Thompson and Dowding (2002:14) action is 'the behaviour following on from a judgement or decision' and Thompson (2002:41) later discusses 'reflection in action'. Here, I shall propose that action is the ongoing dynamic even (and especially) *in* reflection. Therefore, I would rather say 'reflection as action'. The skills for clinical supervision then, are action skills. They are also activity skills. Clinical supervision is an activity in which one is active. It involves active listening to oneself as well as to others. And it involves looking at how arguments and ideas are constructed. There are resources readily available to help us in this latter activity (e.g. Pesut & Herman 1999). How to be active and creative in the clinical supervision process is the principal concern in this chapter.

ACTIVE AWARENESS

What does the adjective *active* describe? Does it refer to a state of:

- being highly activated?
- speaking quickly and loudly?
- making strong and deliberate movements of the body?
- actively listening by forcing eye contact?
- giving strong opinions?
- giving clever insights?
- giving criticism?
- giving praise?

Are these the kinds of activity associated with clinical supervision? Or do they both rather assume and lead to passivity? What do you think? A dozen questions to mull over ... and a few more to follow.

Which of the following statements do you think is 'active' in the context of the clinical supervision relationship ... or might lead to passivity?
- Telling others what you think.
- Problem solving for others.
- Assisting others to develop their own problem-solving skills.
- Telling others how good you think their performance was.
- Telling others how poor you think their performance was.

Perhaps *active*, in clinical supervision, is more to do with an attitude. Is my attitude that of wanting something and then being active in achieving it? The danger is that clinical supervision will always belong to another if I don't own it for myself. If I *let* you supervise me, *allow* you to call the shots, organize the session, choose the questions, then it is rightly yours, not mine. This *fact* is the root of the confusion that some clinicians have about the nature of 'supervision'. If you think that clinical supervision is an onerous task, that you will be exposed to another who will judge or criticize you, then you also think that clinical supervision does not belong to you. You may as well be passive *in* clinical supervision if you think these things. If you were passive would you in fact be having clinical supervision at all? I think not.

Are you waiting for your supervisor to contact you? If so, you are giving away something that rightfully belongs to you!

The notion of being *vigorous* and *active* is suggestive that you actually want something. Some people would call this *desire*. The nature of desire has been widely discussed for at least a century. We are what we desire, say some psychoanalysts. But we can also desire to be passive, to not want. This is somewhat of a paradox. I may not *know* what it is that I desire. Others may know it better than me. They see it on my face; hear it in the ideas that I express. This would be related to Sigmund Freud's challenge to 'unconscious emotion' (Freud 1957:177–179). For Freud, emotions cannot be unconscious even though ideas associated with emotions can be repressed.

My desire is there for all to see, except myself. I may desire to be inactive, for instance. Or, on the other hand, my desire for activity may be blocked or hindered through negative perceptions or experiences. Then again, my desire may be based in an internal removal from myself (Kristeva 1991). I think, however, that we can talk about desire in a more everyday sense. I may not know all the psychological reasons for my desire but I at least know that I would prefer this job over that one — this house, these friends, this country etc. And sometimes I seem to have trouble getting the things that I desire.

In Paris in 1997, while ambling through a maze at the Carousel gardens beside the Louvre, I happened upon *Action enchaînée* (Action in chains), a 1940 bronze statue by Aristide Maillol (1861–1944) and I immediately felt that the artist was on about the same thing. The hands are tied behind the back (I could only see the back) but I saw that the figure is walking forward and propelling the left foot on a mound. Or perhaps preparing to spring forward – also looking to the left almost over the shoulder as if he/she senses a dangerous pass. Perhaps the mound is the edge of a precipice. Perhaps she/he is trying to walk at the edge, feeling for her/his balance. He/she doesn't look too worried, from what I could see of the facial features. Merely contemplative — working out her/his next step, his/her next move. She/he accepts that the hands are tied. The legs are strong and powerful. You will notice here that I have a question about the sex of the figure. I'll return to that question later in the chapter. The important point here, for me, is that the figure wants (desires) to move forward, and does so even when restrained.

Desire is intensely personal, even though others may see my desire better than I see it myself. It is up to each of us to live with her and his desire. To either face it or not face it. This is a choice that can be seen in the ways we act, even if we don't feel that we have choices, or that we are restrained in some way. We need to be actively aware of these factors.

To be active, to notice, in the context of clinical supervision, requires then, that we be receptive. We must be receptive *before* we can be reflective and aware. If we are closed off to possibilities then we won't be able to notice very much at all. So how are we receptive? Well, we are firstly receptive of our professional needs. This is not an easy thing: much of the time we are not even receptive of our personal needs and at times our personal and our professional needs overlap.

My professional need is to listen to my patient. That is, to have the *skill* to listen to my patient. Listening means to be completely attentive: to listen with my ears, but also with my eyes and feelings. I hear the words being spoken; I note the content and the way the words are said. I also see that the patient is acting (doing something) while she or he is speaking. She may be wringing her hands, or shaking her leg. She may be agitated and anxious. So therefore I hear and I look. I also feel. I may feel anxious myself, or bored. I may feel concerned for the patient. I may yawn. Thus, there are physical and emotional states acting themselves out inside and on the surface of my body, just as with the patient. As a professional, however, I have a need *to be able* to listen to the patient at the same time that these states are being played out in/on my own body. Moreover, I may have an associated need not to show that I feel anxious, concerned or bored. And I may be in need of relaxation or time away from the concerns of others. Some professionals find it helpful to keep a record of these needs. The record can be a useful aid in the clinical supervision process.

Keep a notebook in your pocket. During the day, after you have interacted with a patient, note the occasions when you:
■ were thinking about something else (i.e. your mind wandered),
■ became agitated,
■ changed the subject,
■ felt tired or exhausted,
■ looked at your watch or the wall clock,
■ looked out the window,
■ felt happy or sad.

Each of these observations points to your own needs. Clinical supervision will assist you to become actively aware of these needs.

Activity in clinical supervision is at least imaginative. That is, the activity of clinical supervision is one of complex imagery for each of us. We need to think of this imagery as something different from our ordinary thinking activities. For example, it is a very different activity from the thinking we do at the supermarket or at yoga. At the supermarket we process the images that hit us from the shelves (prices, specials, comparisons between brands) at the same time as negotiating the supermarket trolley in congested aisles. At yoga we try to suspend any external world while we allow our thoughts to settle into our sinews and bones. In clinical supervision, we try to bring an element of the external world to our engagement with our supervisor, supervisee or group. That element is the interactive practice in which we were at some time engaged. As supervisees we re-imagine (re-create) the interaction in the clinical supervision space. Thus we start to tell a story of a previous thinking (or imaginative) space. A supervisor will also imagine a previous experience from the story being told by the supervisee (Box 4.1).

BOX 4.1	*Ways in which we can demonstrate active awareness in clinical supervision*
	■ We seek out a supervisor or group
	■ We arrange our clinical supervision time ourselves
	■ We give our complete attention to the session
	■ We reflect on what we are saying or not saying
	■ We welcome the critique of others
	■ We take responsibility for our decision-making
	■ We imagine a past event

CHOICE

One of the essential skills of clinical supervision is to be able to recognize that one has a choice. If one thinks that one has no choice then it is better not to bother with clinical supervision in the first place. Or anything else, for that matter! It is important that we each think carefully through this section ... over to you ...

Some people think we have no choice: that our psychological makeup, our history and our bodies restrict us. Have a look at the following statements:

- Psychologically, some think that we are directed by our unconscious drives and that's the end of the story.
- Historically, or socially, we seem to be formed by our experiences. Our choices then, appear to be connected with what we have learned.
- Physically, it is clear that I don't have any say in my genetic makeup.

Can you think of personal examples in which you did not actively strive or reach out because you felt you were limited in some way with regard to the choices you were able to make? What impact do you think this had on the choices you made? Upon reflection might it be possible to change your perception of these 'limitations'?

Choice is something special, something we need to actively seek out. Something we need to cherish. We speak of choice cuts of beef, for example — there we mean the best. I think it is the same for clinical supervision. Choice itself is the best cut.

Sometimes we forget we have the ability to choose. It is good to remind ourselves, by frequently revisiting the following mantra, that we have a choice:

- I choose ...
- A supervisor or a supervisory group.
- To take responsibility for my clinical supervision.
- To negotiate with my manager.
- To ask for clinical supervision.
- To be on time for my session.
- To say that I agree or don't agree with what is said to me.
- To speak for myself.
- To critique my skills.
- To be open and receptive.
- To accept that I have power.
- To exercise that power in a responsible manner.
- To respect myself.
- To respect the supervisory process.
- To respect my patient/client.

These choices equally apply to the supervisor and the supervisee. Refer to the partnership questionnaires at the end of the chapter to see the results or effects of these choices (Appendixes 1 and 2).

COMMUNICATION AS COLLABORATION

When we speak to others, or relate to them in some other way, we are usually looking for agreement. We want them to understand us and we try to understand them. But sometimes we are too eager in this process. Sometimes we first need to misunderstand each other. In that way we each need to say more about what we mean, or think we mean. Here I shall attempt to say more about what I mean, or think *I mean*, by communication and collaboration.

Philosopher Gilles Deleuze and psychoanalyst Félix Guattari (1994) try to locate the space of philosophy as creation of concepts. Since I believe that we are all philosophers, and I agree with them about creation, I think all of us can be creative in our work with our concepts. One of the products of creation, they say, is communication, although communication, for them, is not in itself creative.

They tell us that communication creates consensus (Deleuze & Guattari 1994:6). What this means, to me, is that when we speak to each other and understand (or misunderstand) each other we are consenting to a process. We may even agree to disagree but even that is a consensus — as is the very disagreement itself. The very fact of communicating with someone (being there and speaking or listening to them) is a consensus. When we speak words to each other we agree upon a meaning of the words, even if we don't agree with what's being said. This is another form of consensus.

Communication is an acceptance that we are social beings. Being social beings means that we exist together and share common characteristics, language, some values, some perspectives and many disagreements.

When you disagree with someone, are you still communicating? What are you communicating?

Do you agree that there is a consensus implied in both the process of communication and the words we use together? If you think there is, how would you explain this consensus to another person? If you don't agree, how would you explain your position?

Do you think that communication can be creative? How?

What is the difference between communication with yourself and communicating with another person?

Do you think that disagreeing with someone is a form of consensus? Or do you think that this would be a contradiction in terms? Try to explore the reasons for your conclusion.

Clinical supervision brings together clinicians and patients in a very particular way. When a clinician is having clinical supervision, what is discussed is the relationship with a patient. The clinician doesn't focus on the patient, but rather focuses on herself or himself. Supervision is about the clinician's side of the relationship. It looks at the skills of the clinician via an examination of what is said, what is not said; what is felt, what is not felt; what is done (acted), what is not done.

When I talk to a patient there are at least two kinds of reflection that I engage in. I reflect back to the patient what I hear her/him say and I reflect back on myself to ensure that I am fully engaged in the relationship. For example, the patient may say to me: 'I feel sad today. I don't think I can go out and do the shopping.' Now, there are a number of responses I can make to this statement:

- I can say nothing. This is a reflection to the patient of silence.

- 'You feel sad today?' This is a reflection of the first part of the patient's statement — and asks for more information.

- 'You feel sad today.' This is a reflection of acknowledgement.

- 'You need to shop.' This is a reflection of direction. It bypasses the feelings of the patient (but doesn't diminish them) and homes in on a necessary physical activity.

- 'Does feeling sad prevent you from going out?' This is a suggestive reflection and links two ideas.

- 'Yes, it's hard to shop when you're feeling sad.' This is a suggestive interpretation.

There are more possibilities but these six reflections demonstrate the point. It will take the second mode of reflection (reflection back on self) for the clinician to gain an understanding of where the reflective statements are coming from and upon which clinical principles they are based. There is no clinical point in responding to a patient unless one simultaneously examines the response. Otherwise, I may as well say anything at all. This simultaneous examination is practised in clinical supervision.

We see then that there are a couple of collaborations going on. First, one collaborates with the patient to try to come to some understanding or consensus of things. Then one collaborates with oneself to gain some understanding of the clinical nature of one's skills. Later, in supervision, one collaborates with the supervisor or group. Here, there is an equivalent or *parallel process* in play where the original interaction is repeated and re-reflected (see Fox 1989 for a full discussion and references for parallel process).

DIFFERENCE AND SIMILARITY

Patients deserve to receive a highly skilled service from health professionals. This requires that clinicians constantly strive to understand the communicative processes in which they are engaged. When clinicians overly introduce their own feelings, opinions and values into an interaction it could be suggested that they prevent patients from exploring what is important for them. Not everyone will agree with me here. Some will say that clinicians can only present themselves in their feelings, opinions and values. But the question I then ask myself is how the patient's perspective comes to be truly valued.

The dilemma of this question may never be resolved. It can, however, and should be addressed in clinical supervision because it is a dilemma about boundaries. How much of myself is it appropriate to introduce to a patient? It is equally important to recognize that I may not be the same every day, or even on the same day. We might hear a resonance in this sentiment of Michel Foucault's famous maxim: 'Do not ask who I am and do not ask me to remain the same' (cited in Dreyfus & Rabinow 1982:xiv). However, this is only to caution us in being too comfortable with what we think we know of others, the world and ourselves. Of course I am the same person, but in so far as I am constantly *refinding* and *refining* myself in my experiences I can never really be quite the same. Each new experience, each new association will make me slightly different from the person I was prior to those experiences and associations.

Recently I heard an excellent paper where cultural supervision was discussed (Westerman 2004). There, I became more acutely aware of the importance of cultural differences *vis-à-vis* Aboriginal societies. Although I had been aware of these differences before, I now came to see that there were many cultural subtleties that require a specialist knowledge and approach. Usually, I have a removed or intellectual knowledge of other cultures. There is, however, another kind of knowledge, that can only develop when one has direct and deep experience of another cultural group. Cultural groups can be ethnic groups, or groups we sometimes refer to as sub-cultures.

Think of a time when you were confronted with your own lack of knowledge or understanding of the intricacies of another cultural group. What was going on? How would you discuss this as an issue in clinical supervision? What if those same cultural issues were also present in clinical supervision?

BOX 4.2	*What it means to say that we are the same and/or different from others*

- We are the same as others
- We are different from others
- Our patients are like us and not like us
- We are similar yet different from our supervisor/ee
- We are not the quite same each day/year
- Neither is anyone else always quite the same
- We don't 'automatically' understand another's perspective

PROXIMITY — GETTING CLOSE — BUT NOT TOO CLOSE

Here we can consider for ourselves issues pertaining to proximity in supervision: fear, warmth and resistance. This description will allow us to examine, as if with a microscope, the dynamics in which we constantly find ourselves. By analysing these dynamics we may be able to go some way in assisting newer clinicians to feel the benefits of clinical supervision at both a personal and a professional level. The closeness we have in supervision can be seen in parallel with the closeness we have with our patients. Each of us has a different way of getting close and each of us is different in how close we get. It is good to consider what all this means for ourselves.

I once had a patient whom I regularly saw in her home. She was 80 years of age, had a lovely garden and house and cooked me biscuits and other nice things. She had a family but they rarely visited. I was so comfortable with her that I didn't notice how much I liked seeing her. I looked forward to our appointments. At Christmas she gave me a lovely gift and I reciprocated. I was 'up front' with the team about these things and no one seemed too concerned because of her age. However, it gradually dawned on me, through clinical supervision, that my needs were being met at her expense. I needed to see her more than she needed to see me. Once I came to this realization I was able to discuss with her a more professional plan for future visits. I learned from this experience that sometimes we become the patients, and our patients the therapists.

Think about the people you get close to. How close do you get? What do you think are the reasons for this? Write these reasons down and refer back to them from time to time to see whether your position changes with different experiences.

BOX 4.3	*Ways in which to get close and yet keep our distance*

- We respect boundaries — our own and those of others as well as those that join/separate us
- We accept that others see and hear us
- We accept that we are similar yet different
- We have control over what we reveal
- We have control over what we accept
- We actively notice the space(s) between ourselves and others

A PARTNERSHIP OF REFLECTION

Partnership is a form of friendship. That is, when we form partnerships we get close to one another (more or less), share our thoughts and/or feelings, extend ourselves to another person or persons. To truly reflect with another person we connect with them in a very personal way. The expression, 'I am there for you' is very apt here. Where is 'there'? It is in the place in which I am needed: 'there', to share the pain, hopes or thoughts.

Reminders

An important skill in the clinical supervision process is being able to bring together the things we want to review and reflect upon. We recollect, or remind ourselves of what it was that occurred in an interaction. Ludwig Wittgenstein remarks: 'Something that we know when no one asks us, but no longer know

BOX 4.4

Reflection, in the origin of the word, is related to bending back (Brown 1993). There are several elements of reflection that are worth noting and considering:

- I can reflect outwardly and I can reflect inwardly

- When you say something to me I can say it back to you. This is outward reflection

- When I say something and think about what I have just said, this is inward reflection; so too when you say something to me and I think about what you have said

- When we expose our thoughts together this is group reflection. This is not an easy thing to achieve (see Chapter 8)

when we are supposed to give an account of it, is something that we need to *remind* ourselves of. (And it is obviously something of which for some reason it is difficult to remind oneself)' (Wittgenstein 1967: remark 89). This process is quite involved, for as we all know, our memory sometimes plays tricks on us. And our memory consists of images, both visual and verbal, at least, and sometimes emotional. To complicate things further, sometimes we need to be reminded about other elements of memory. I was recently reminded, in hearing a paper by Tania Yegdich (Yegdich 2005), that for Freud, our memories are revealed in our actions. The past is repeated in our bodies, though we don't normally recognize it (Freud, 1958). That is to say, other people see our memories (better than we do) just as they see our emotions. For Marcel Proust, we can recapture our memories through a sensory experience (e.g. smell) or an action (e.g. tripping). These events can remind us (repeat for us) something from our deep past. For Proust then, they help us to regain those memories we thought we had lost (Proust 1983).

My primary reminder in clinical supervision is that it is about saying and hearing — this implies both verbal exposure and concentration. Those primarily listening in a clinical supervision session form images of what is being said — like pictures of that which is heard described. And the other senses are also in operation. For instance, the listeners see the person who is speaking, so the images they form for themselves are informed by the sense of sight as well. These listeners are also influenced by their own life experiences. But the more important picture is that formed of *self* by each person involved in the clinical supervision process. The more I sense another the more I sense myself.

First then, I remind myself of what clinical supervision is and is not. It is different for different people. For many of us it is a critical reflection on self, on the words we say or do not say to patients, the actions we do and do not do. For many, clinical supervision is not performance management, case management, or therapy (Yegdich 1999), although it may be closely aligned with these practices. Secondly, I remind myself of the need for clinical supervision. No one except myself can effect a self-critique for me (in this sense I am ultimately my own supervisor). It is up to each of us. If we don't do it then we could say that we don't know who we are as clinicians. Thirdly, I remind myself of what self-critique is in a clinical setting. It does not mean that I exist alone. It cannot mean that, for the *clinical* implies more than one person. I exist for the patient (in so far as she or he is a patient) and the patient exists for me (in so far as I am a clinician).

The clinical setting, of course, implies more than one clinician or profession. It implies a number of professions, at least, to which each of us belongs, and from which we derive our professional identities. Davies (2002:32) discusses the way that professional identities are often formed in a negative relation to others. However, professions can also complement each other in a positive way. They can operate alongside each other: co-operate. In the clinical setting then, I exist as a clinician among other similar clinicians and other professions. The patient needs to be confident that I don't work and speak alone — off my own bat, so to speak. In the sense that we do speak as clinicians, we do have to be seen to have credentials. We are granted our professional status by various bodies. We need to remind ourselves of this. We have a commitment to the codes of our various professions. Self-critique takes this into account.

The context of clinical supervision then, is one of reminders. What now can we say it is that constitutes the reminders within clinical supervision? I am having clinical supervision with another or others. They may be from my own profession or they may be from other professions. This other, or these others, assist me to remind myself of my clinical skills and the manner in which I employ them.

I need to remind myself that the patient is multifaceted. That is, that she and he are not one element, not one set of symptoms or concerns, not existing alone. She and he have a family, friends, and a network. I, as a clinician, am part of that network: someone special to whom this person confides personal information, sometimes intensely personal. When a patient confides in those considered professional she or he trusts that they are knowledgeable; that they will draw from their experience in listening to issues and guide, or thoughtfully sit alongside, the patient towards the resolution sought for. The patient also has a history, a childhood, a cultural connection, desires and fears. We must remind ourselves of this.

And I must remind myself that I too am multifaceted. Thus, I must remind myself that I am interacting with the patient from my own complex perspective. We all know critical elements that constitute that perspective: our beliefs, values, knowledge, and physical and emotional states. These are elements we often take for granted in our day-to-day interactions with patients and colleagues. This reminder about myself is an ongoing activity; something that needs to be practised every day. I need to check myself, so to speak, to see how I am feeling: am I tired, hung-over, concerned about my finances, or my close personal relationships? Do I have a headache? These are some of the physical and emotional elements. And then, what of my beliefs? That is, my beliefs about myself as a professional — my skills and abilities. Are my beliefs in line with my actual skills and abilities, or are they under- or over-estimated? This reminding requires me to re-evaluate my knowledge. Closely aligned with my beliefs are my values.

My values underpin all my judgements and assessments. When the patient tells me he or she has beaten his or her partner in an alcoholic fury I am immediately attuned to my own experiences of violence. I react in a certain way to this information. I am either critical and show it, or critical and try not to show it, or non-critical and try to comprehend the broader context of the life of the person who sits opposite me. Each of these attitudes has consequences. There are consequences for the person opposite me, just as there are consequences for myself.

The person may feel victimized, lied to, listened to. She or he may proceed to trust or not to trust me. The consequences for myself may be that I feel scandalized, torn between conflicting interests/feelings, or comfortable in the knowledge that I am utilizing my professional listening skills in the most objective way. I can only achieve this objectivity by reminding myself that I may not have heard the patient in her or his own terms.

This listening, then, is not passive. As I listen, I seek to understand, to clinically interpret the information. This is a form of assessment, evaluation or judgement in a positive sense. But how do I ensure the objectivity? First, I look for the objective signs that my clinical texts have alerted me to (Nagelkerk 2001:24). I try for an objective assessment of the person's physical and emotional state and sometimes of her or his mental state. These are objective signs, surely, that everyone may see — and see in the way they have been taught to observe. And, at the same time, I must be objective to myself.

This then is a basic but powerful reminder. The patient is not a passive recipient and neither am I. She and he have needs beyond the ones we ordinarily identify as health professionals (usually physical and psychological). There are other more basic needs to do with social connection. One might suggest that these needs form the very nexus of a society: perhaps we could call them communicative needs. Communication, while often taken for granted, also implies masks and barriers. We often hide (and/or try to hide) ourselves rather than to reveal ourselves in what is popularly termed a 'transparent' or 'overt' fashion (Jourard 1971). This human facility of hiding ourselves is common knowledge to all of us. Therefore, it is easy to see that we also have the concurrent facility of attempting to uncover the hidden. Think about what you may want to hide from others. Also think about how you might try to uncover the hidden. What are the social conventions around both of these activities? That is, what do we need to keep in mind when we seek to hide, on the one hand, or seek to know, on the other?

Review

One of the elements of reflection is review. Review is re-view. We look again — do a double take. And just as listening also includes looking and feeling, so too does review include all these elements. To look back, is to repeat, to re-live. Thus, in clinical supervision, we repeat the experience we had with our patient. There is of course one element that may appear to be missing: the patient. This is why it is so important to bring the patient's words and actions to the session. We can't have clinical supervision if there is no patient–clinician interaction involved. There is a recipient of our skills and that recipient must be included (Yegdich 1999). The focus, however, is not on the patient, but on the *interaction*, in which the patient is an *essential element*.

Review does not end at the clinical supervision session. I now need to go on and review my supervision activity. I need to actively do this. Winstanley and White (2003) provide us with useful directions in this activity. We should, however, work out for ourselves just what it is that we will review in terms of our clinical supervision.

Go to a quiet place by yourself and think about the following. It might aid your reflections to make some notes:

- What would it feel like to constantly reflect on what we are saying or doing?
- When we give ongoing feedback to our peers/supervisor/supervisee, how is this both a constant process and an intermittent process?
- How do we demonstrate our commitment to others in the clinical supervision relationship?
- How is clinical supervision itself a review? How do we review all of our varied commitments?
- How would you tell yourself about the changes you have made to your interactive practices?
- If there were someone with you now, how would you be thinking and speaking about these issues? Would it make a difference if the person came from another culture or social sub-group or was a different sex or had a different sexual orientation from yours? How would it make a difference?
- What might be the implications for you in clinical supervision of reflecting on the above?

Repetition

We talked about repeating ourselves in the previous section on review. We saw how review included reflection. Now we see how repetition includes review. Repetition is about doing or saying again (and again we are reminded of Freud). In clinical supervision repetition is an important clue as to what is important to us. Thus I might find myself saying much the same thing but in four different ways:

'I just wasn't able to get close to that patient'
'I felt that there was no connection between us'
'There was a distance between us'
'I couldn't start up a conversation'

It is important to become skilled in:

1) hearing, and
2) reflecting these repetitions.

For we must also hear and reflect to our patients the repetitions we hear from them. Clinical supervision assists us to become more attuned to these repetitions.

BOX 4.5

Reminding ourselves of factors to do with repetition:

- We repeat ourselves (say twice or more)
- We repeat our processes (do twice and more)
- We never reach the end
- We repeat (tell) what occurred in the patient interaction (parallel process both ways)

BOX 4.5	*(cont'd)*

- We repeat (reflect) what we hear
- Our problems repeat themselves
- Our answers (and questions) repeat themselves

I often find that I constantly raise the same problem or concern in clinical supervision. For example, I once looked after a depressed patient who lived at home on his own. I thought about him quite regularly. I knew his family rarely visited and I knew that he found it difficult to look after his little dog. I looked forward to seeing him and playing with the dog. We would talk about his war experiences and all the exciting things he had done in his life. This is a form of reminiscence therapy. However, I came to see through clinical supervision, that the reminiscence therapy was more for me than for him. The conversations were similar to those I had had with my own grandfather. I also saw that I was repeating a pattern of having my own needs met at the expense of those of the patient. I needed to see him more than he needed to see me.

Professionally I needed to (re)learn from this experience that sometimes we become the patients, and our patients the therapists. What about yourself? Do you find that certain issues or approaches tend to repeat themselves?

AN INTERIM CONCLUSION: LETTING OUR QUESTIONS STAND?

Michèle Le Dœuff tells us: 'For fifteen years [Vladimir] Jankélévitch was my very kind supervisor and friend. My youth owes a great deal to his liberalism and benevolence. ... Like Simone de Beauvoir, he left me with my questions' (Le Dœuff 1991:352). Now, Le Dœuff is talking about another kind of supervision here, more to do with patronage. But in so far as we are all questioners the quote is apt. To be left with our questions is something Le Dœuff encourages; these questions belong to us, after all, not to someone else. Clinical supervision is about someone else hearing our questions and showing us how these questions have been heard, but certainly not answering them for us. It is as though we stand face to face with another in clinical supervision while at the same time standing face to face with our questions.

What does it mean to say that we stand face to face with another in clinical supervision? For Michèle Le Dœuff we stand before others in order to give them a good hearing. We don't block them by too easily thinking that we understand them. To give someone a good hearing takes some time. This is why we should not abandon our clinical supervision if, as a supervisee, we think we are not immediately or correctly heard, or if, as a supervisor, we think we can't immediately or correctly hear. On the contrary, these *mishearings* should give us confidence

BOX 4.6	*Reminders of where our questions stand*

- Where the questions are asked
- Well clear of an answer
- With us — we don't give them away
- In relation to a patient?
- In relation to ourselves?

that we are on the right track. For it would mean that we are not rushing to conclusions.

One reason that we need to let our questions stand in clinical supervision is that they are *our* questions. No one can answer them but we ourselves. As Sidney M Jourard tells us: 'In a certain sense, every person is an animated questionnaire. Each of us embodies a whole batch of questions that we address to everyone whom we contact' (Jourard 1971:11). If someone else answers your questions then the answers belong with them, and their questions are not likely to be exactly the same as yours. Another reason we let them stand is that the questions and the answers constantly shift or change. And some questions imply answers. To take my earlier example of the bronze statue near the Louvre in Paris, the question as to the sex of the figure is my question, a question I may not need to answer let alone ask. For the question may not be mine alone but may be a question based in my engagement as a social being at this particular moment in history. I may choose not to ask or answer the question just because I don't yet know all the conditions that have prompted me to want (desire) to raise the question in the first place. We see then just how complex the matter is. In clinical supervision I must be constantly aware of what it is that I may be asking, the context in which I am asking it, and the implications of an answer. By the way, I did happen across a picture of the statue and now know its sex and history. The question I still have though is how the figure so confidently strides forward while having its hands tied behind its back. My question. Perhaps this is the question I take with me into every clinical supervision session. Is this a way, then, in which communication can be creative? To let our questions stand — before another?

Today I might wonder if I over-reacted to a comment made by my patient. I might think: 'Was I provoked into making a sarcastic remark to the patient?' (The implied answer is 'Yes!') Tomorrow, however, I might think: 'I didn't over-react, I responded appropriately given the circumstances.' But I can't leave it there. I need to examine my response and the effect it may have had on both the patient and myself. In six months' time I might have an entirely different question. For example: 'What are the conditions whereby I might be less than professional in my interactions with my patients?' There is no implied answer here — the question merely calls for a description and a creative understanding.

On reflection ... chapter summary

- A supervisory partnership is an active event which needs constant work.
- To be active implies being receptive and collaborative.
- Clinical supervision is about saying and hearing.
- An essential skill in the clinical supervision relationship is being able to remind ourselves of a number of important factors, the most important of which is that we have choices to do with how we hear, how we reflect and how we ask questions of ourselves and others.
- Reflection is inward to ourselves and outward to others. Others also reflect back to us.

Let's flip back to the jumble we had at the beginning of the chapter (Figure 4.1). Compare with Figure 4.2. Hopefully our thoughts are a little more organized; the pieces fitting together into a coherent whole. There is, however, no perfect fit: something is always left over. But we need to keep striving, in partnership, for the best possible fit. The following questionnaires can help us in this endeavour and also act as reminders of our flourishing and ongoing roles in the clinical supervision partnership. And a final question around roles: just who is the supervisee and who is the supervisor? Can we be both at the same time? I'm asking you. But am I expecting you to answer for me? Perhaps you will have other questions.

FURTHER READING

Cutcliffe J R, Butterworth T, Proctor B (eds) 2001 Fundamental themes in clinical supervision. Routledge, London, UK

Fish D, Twinn S 1997 Quality clinical supervision in the health care professions. Butterworth-Heinemann, Oxford, UK

Kaiser T L 1997 Supervisory relationships: exploring the human element. Brooks/Cole, Pacific Grove, USA

Nicholls D, Mitchell-Dawson B 2002 Promoting mental health in nurses through clinical supervision. In: Morrow L, Verins I, Willis E (eds) Mental health and work: issues and perspectives. VicHealth and Auseinet, Flinders University, Adelaide, Australia. Online. Available at: http://www.auseinet.com/resources/auseinet/mhw/index.php

Yegdich T 1998 How not to do clinical supervision in nursing. Journal of Advanced Nursing 28(1):198–202

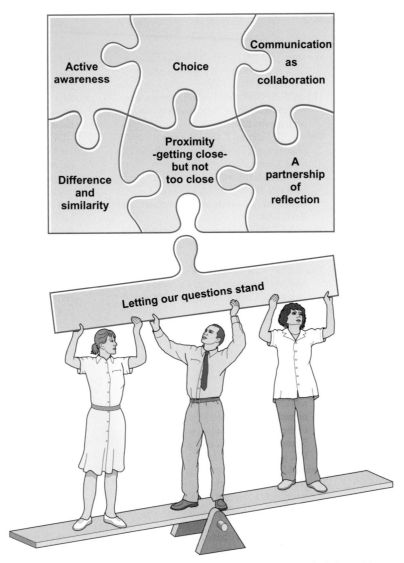

Figure 4.2 Returning to the puzzle of the supervisory relationship — getting the balance right

REFERENCES

Brown L (ed) 1993 The new shorter Oxford English dictionary on historical principles. Clarendon, Oxford, UK

Davies C 2002 Managing identities: workers, professions and identity. Nursing Management 9(5):31–36

Deleuze G, Guattari F 1994 What is philosophy? (Burchell G & Tomlinson H, trans.) Verso, London, UK

Dreyfus H L, Rabinow P 1982 Michel Foucault: beyond structuralism and Hermeneutics. Harvester Wheatsheaf, New York, USA

Driscoll J 2002 Practising clinical supervision: a reflective approach. Elsevier Science, Oxford, UK

Fox R 1989 Relationship: the cornerstone of clinical supervision social casework. Journal of Contemporary Social Work (March):146–152

Freud S 1957 The unconscious. In: Strachey J (ed) Papers on metapsychology [1915]: the standard edition of the complete psychological works of Sigmund Freud, XIV. Hogarth, London, UK, p 159–215

Freud S 1958 Remembering, repeating and working-through. In: Strachey J (ed) Papers on technique [1914]: the standard edition of the complete psychological works of Sigmund Freud, XII. Hogarth, London, UK, p 147–156

Jourard S M 1971 The transparent self. D Van Nostrand, New York, USA

Kristeva J 1991 Strangers to ourselves. (Leon S Roudiez, trans.) Columbia University, New York, USA

Le Dœuff M 1991 Hipparchia's choice: an essay concerning women, philosophy, etc. (Selous T, trans.) Blackwell, Oxford, UK

Nagelkerk J 2001 Diagnostic reasoning: case analysis in primary care practice. W B Saunders, Philadelphia, USA

Pesut D J, Herman J 1999 Clinical reasoning: the art and science of critical and creative thinking. Delmar Publishers, New York, USA

Proust M 1983 Remembrance of things past. (Scott Moncrieff C K, Kilmartin T, trans.) Penguin, London, UK

Thompson C 2002 Human error, bias, decision making and judgement in nursing. In: Thompson C, Dowding D (eds) Clinical decision making and judgement in nursing. Churchill Livingstone, London, UK

Thompson C, Dowding D 2002 Clinical decision making and judgement in nursing: an introduction. In: Thompson C, Dowding D (eds) Clinical decision making and judgement in nursing. Churchill Livingstone, London, UK

Westerman T 2004 The value of unique service provision for Aboriginal people – the benefits of starting from scratch. The Mental Health Services Conference Inc. of Australia and New Zealand, 1–3 September

Winstanley J, White E 2003 Clinical supervision: models, measures and best practice. Nurse Researcher 10(4):7–22

Wittgenstein L 1967 Philosophical investigations. 3rd edn. (Anscombe G E M, trans.) Blackwell, Oxford, UK

Yegdich T 1999 Lost in the crucible of supportive clinical supervision: supervision is not therapy. Journal of Advanced Nursing 29(5):1265–1275

Yegdich T 2005 Remembering, repeating and working through. Clinical Supervision Conference, Cape Shanck, Australia

| APPENDIX 1 | *Partnership Questionnaire for Supervisee* |

For each of the following statements mark an **X** on the line to indicate where you see yourself situated. *(Try to do this exercise every 3 months. Photocopy the page.)*

Of course it will open up a dialogue if both parties in clinical supervision complete this independently and bring it along to the next session as a discussion item to validate the partnership.

I take responsibility for my clinical supervision

(always)   *(somewhere in between)*   *(never)*

_____

I feel comfortable to negotiate with my manager around my clinical supervision needs

(always)   *(somewhere in between)*   *(never)*

_____

I feel comfortable to ask for clinical supervision

(always)   *(somewhere in between)*   *(never)*

_____

I can tell my supervisor that I don't agree with what is said to me

(always)   *(somewhere in between)*   *(never)*

_____

I know how to critique my skills

(always)   *(somewhere in between)*   *(never)*

_____

I am open and receptive

(always)   *(somewhere in between)*   *(never)*

_____

I accept that I have power in the clinical supervision relationship

(always)   *(somewhere in between)*   *(never)*

_____

I exercise my power in a responsible manner

(always)   *(somewhere in between)*   *(never)*

_____

I respect the supervisory process

(always)   *(somewhere in between)*   *(never)*

_____

| APPENDIX 2 | *Partnership Questionnaire for Supervisor* |

For each of the following statements mark an **X** on the line to indicate where you see yourself situated. *(Try to do this exercise every 3 months. Photocopy the page.)*

Of course it will open up a dialogue if both parties in clinical supervision complete this independently and bring it along to the next session as a discussion item to validate the partnership.

I respect the responsibility that the supervisee owns for her/his clinical supervision

(always)   *(somewhere in between)*   *(never)*

_____

I am comfortable with the supervisee leading the negotiations around session times

(always)   *(somewhere in between)*   *(never)*

_____

I am aware that the supervisee has control of the problem-solving process

(always)   *(somewhere in between)*   *(never)*

_____

I can tell the supervisee that I don't agree with what is said to me

(always)   *(somewhere in between)*   *(never)*

_____

I receive supervision myself

(always)   *(somewhere in between)*   *(never)*

_____

I am open and receptive

(always)   *(somewhere in between)*   *(never)*

_____

I accept that I have power in the clinical supervision relationship

(always)   *(somewhere in between)*   *(never)*

_____

I exercise my power in a responsible manner

(always)   *(somewhere in between)*   *(never)*

_____

I respect the supervisory process

(always)   *(somewhere in between)*   *(never)*

_____

SUPERVISORY METHODS AND APPROACHES

5

Psychological approaches to the clinical supervision encounter

Graham Sloan

INTRODUCTION

I started my registered mental nurse (RMN) modular training in 1982. Clinical supervision (CS) was something I did not experience until 1986 when I took up the post of staff nurse (SN) in an adult psychotherapy day hospital. A psychoanalyst working in the unit delivered CS in a group format, and all staff had to participate. As far as I can recall, there was a great deal of conflict among some members of the team and this animosity would seep into supervision. On reflection, supervision was used to contain team dynamics and provide an opportunity to explore staff relations; client-related issues were rarely discussed. I was uncertain of what I should be doing in the group meetings, since being relatively new to the team I did not have any tensions with my colleagues.

Around the same period, the charge nurse (CN) started to provide individual CS to the nursing staff in the unit. At that time, CS had not stimulated much interest and there was a distinct lack of conceptual analysis and empirical research on CS and its relevance to nursing in the United Kingdom. I did not receive any training in CS, and nor was I given the option not to participate. I was informed that CS would give me an opportunity to discuss my work with clients and anything that was of concern. Being a new member to the team, I had much enthusiasm for my work, wanted to fit in and create a good impression with my colleagues and line manager. At that time, I understood CS as a 'must do' activity and that it was provided by the CN, my line manager.

I recall talking about two clients. The first was a middle-aged woman whom I was seeing on an individual basis. She had experienced a difficult, abusive childhood and relationship difficulties were a common occurrence. She was depressed, had been an inpatient on many occasions and was considered at risk of harming herself. She had tried to kill herself on many occasions. My enthusiasm in wanting to help was particularly strong and I wanted to ensure her safety; I made myself more accessible with this woman than with my other clients and sometimes the fifty-minute sessions would extend to well over an hour. I took this to supervision hoping that I would be able to explore my reactions. My supervisor praised my efforts and thought that I was providing good nursing care. Having the approval of my line manager was important and so his comments were reassuring. None the less, I remained perplexed and uncertain of my reactions when working with this client.

The second client I recall also suffered from depression. He had been in and out of psychiatric hospitals for most of his adult life; he had seen numerous psychiatrists, therapists, CPNs and clinical psychologists. Throughout the several sessions we had, despite conveying motivation for change, asking for help, the client was always reluctant to engage in working on ideas that had emerged during his sessions. In addition to feeling deskilled, I found myself irritated, confused and critical of his inability to take things forward. Following my presentation of these issues, my supervisor suggested I discharge this client since he wasn't making progress. My supervisor thought that if the client had been unable to progress with the level and range of previous interventions, it was unlikely that I would achieve anything. The client was discharged from the unit and community follow-up arranged. I felt further deskilled but also sensed that I had let this client down.

I have had many positive experiences with CS since my initial introduction. Its delivery has ranged between individual, group and triadic formats. Nursing staff who had undergone psychotherapy training have provided some of these experiences and at other times CS has been provided by a psychiatrist, clinical psychologist or occupational therapist. I would argue that consistent provision of CS has assisted me in achieving a high standard of care. Intuitively, I would argue that the care I have provided to clients has benefited from my commitment to CS. Together with other professional development strategies, consistent engagement with CS has progressed my professional competence. However, it has also had other significant benefits which are not as easily evidenced or appreciated.

As I alluded to earlier, engaging in a helping relationship is not always an easy or straightforward activity. Supervision has enabled me to tolerate my uncertainties when working with particular clients and helped identify ways of working which have been positive for my clients, but which I have not always immediately acknowledged. It has assisted me in developing confidence in my provision of clients' care and has guided me towards appreciating unhelpful ways of working and supporting new ways of relating with clients. In these contexts, in addition to CS being didactic and cognitive, it has facilitated the working through of emotional material inextricably associated with my clinical work.

It is my belief that the therapeutic relationship and the delivery of helpful interventions is an important focus for CS for a broad range of healthcare professionals, occupational therapists, physiotherapists, and general nurses, for example. Throughout their professional careers, all healthcare professionals are expected to engage with clients in an intentionally helpful manner; ease clients' suffering by dealing with a heavy burden of emotional distress. In this chapter I provide an overview of some of the conceptual models of CS, which facilitate detailed exploration of the supervisee's relations with clients. Following on from this, I highlight some of the key issues pertaining to the CS encounter. But before proceeding further it is necessary to clarify the perspective of CS referred to in this chapter.

 How important do you think it might be as an individual practitioner to think of your own patients and clients in a 'psychological' way in the clinical supervision situation? If not in clinical supervision, where else do you discuss this aspect of your work?

PSYCHOLOGICAL PERSPECTIVE OF CLINICAL SUPERVISION

CS is considered to be an essential requirement for learning and professional development within the professions working with individuals. It is not a novel concept within psychotherapy, counselling, clinical psychology and social work. On the contrary, it has a well-established position and is now generally recognized as a means of developing practitioners' therapeutic integrity (Bernard & Goodyear 1998, Doehrmann 1976, Holloway & Neufeldt 1995, Kilminster & Jolly 2000, Loganbill et al 1982, Watkins 1990).

Loganbill et al (1982:4) defined supervision as:

> An intensive, interpersonally focused, one-to-one relationship in which one person is designated to facilitate the development of therapeutic competence in the other person.

It is widely recognized in psychotherapy communities that engaging therapeutically, in what is essentially a helping relationship, with clients is complicated and demanding. Psychotherapy is a human encounter. During therapy, an interpersonal system involving client and therapist exists; both must be understood in this context. The client cannot be understood in therapy independent of the therapist. The therapist has his own human peculiarities and sensitivities which will inevitably interact with those of the client; the therapist contributes to what transpires during therapy (Safran & Segal 1996). Tania Yegdich, a nurse psychotherapist trained in psychoanalytic psychotherapy, illuminated this important focus for nurses:

> The nature of clinical supervision has as its narrative, the patient's human suffering. What is examined in supervision is the effect of the patient's suffering on the nurse's ability to respond, interact and to think.
> Yegdich, 1996:95

CS provides an opportunity for the supervisee to consider their contribution to the therapeutic relationship. It facilitates exploration of how they intervene during their attempts at resolving clients' psychological suffering, encouraging them to evaluate the impact of such ways of being. Furthermore, it provides a forum where the supervisee may contemplate their own emotional reactions, which are inherent in this work. CS represents an opportunity for practitioners to develop their competence in, and contribution towards, this therapeutic endeavour.

As in therapy, during CS it is the client's needs, rather than those of the supervisee, which are prioritized. Essentially, CS is an educational opportunity where the supervisee can develop their competence in interacting with those with whom they are engaged in a helping relationship. Ultimately, it is the supervisee's clients who will benefit. Conversely, during therapy, the person in receipt of this process (client) is assisted towards alleviation of their psychological distress.

- Read Yegdich's paper 'Lost in a crucible of supportive clinical supervision: supervision is not therapy' published in the Journal of Advanced Nursing (Yegdich 1999).
- What might be the consequences of CS having a focus on the psychological wellbeing of the supervisee rather than that of their clients?
- If focused discussion regarding clients does not take place during CS, where does it happen?
- What might the consequences of a practitioner not considering the therapeutic relationship in clinical supervision be?
- Think back over your last two clinical supervision sessions … what were the key items you discussed? How much of what you discussed in clinical supervision placed much importance on the helping relationship between you and your patient/client?

It is hoped that the reader will be excited by this perspective on CS and will gain knowledge and insights about some of the psychologically focused conceptual frameworks for CS.

CONCEPTUAL FRAMEWORKS FOR CLINICAL SUPERVISION

There are two main categories of supervision model, psychotherapy-based models and supervision-specific models. Psychotherapy-based models use the assumptions, methods and techniques of a particular orientation to psychotherapy to guide CS, for example, psychodynamic approaches. The second category of models are developed specifically for supervision and training and include, for example, developmental models. It is beyond the scope of this chapter to attempt to describe all the available psychotherapy-based models so only a few have been selected. Similarly, it is beyond the scope of the present chapter to describe supervision-based models outlined by Faugier and Butterworth (1994), Hawkins and Shohet (2000), Proctor (1987), and Van Ooijen (2000).

It is my intention to provide readers with an overview of:

- cognitive therapy (CT) supervision,
- supervision guided by Heron's six category intervention analysis,
- solution-focused (SF) supervision.

These frameworks have been selected for a number of reasons, but mainly because of their practical utility in the clinical supervision situation. In my view they offer a useful structure for adopting in sessions, are relatively easy to learn by a diverse range of practitioners not engaged in mental health work, and most importantly, present the real possibility of evaluating the effectiveness of clinical supervision.

What informs your supervision currently whether as a supervisor or supervisee? Think about and/or arrange to formally discuss in your next clinical supervision session what model(s) underpins its delivery. Who decided what model guides your supervision and why? How do you know if it is working?

COGNITIVE THERAPY SUPERVISION

Supervision, which is provided using the CT model, is similar to the therapy process in that it aims to be focused, structured, educational and collaborative. However, as Newman (1998:105) stressed, 'clinical supervision is not psychotherapy'. None the less, it is acknowledged that the practice of supervisor and supervisee (within and between supervision) will be influenced by their own core beliefs, underlying assumptions and automatic thoughts. Supervision using this framework has as its focus the development of the supervisee's therapeutic work. The supervisory encounter is structured using a supervision agreement (Howard 1997) and each session is structured by an agenda, and in the same way that CT aims to make links across sessions, CT supervision aims to summarize previous session content and review any learning which has occurred between sessions. An example of a CT supervision session agenda is outlined in Box 5.1 based on the work of Liese and Beck (1997:121).

Todd and Freshwater (1999) and Sloan and colleagues (2000) highlighted the usefulness of this psychotherapy supervision framework, first described by Padesky (1996) and Liese and Beck (1997), for nursing. While Todd and Freshwater (1999) illustrated the similarities between reflective practice and guided discovery, Sloan and colleagues (2000) clarified that while the approach was devised to help develop the therapeutic competence of cognitive therapists, its use in nursing contexts merit consideration. The cognitive therapy supervision framework, by addressing both the processes and content of supervision, highlights its essential purpose, the development of the supervisee's therapeutic competence. Consequently, its relevance to other healthcare professionals seems obvious, particularly since those healthcare professionals who are in direct contact with patients will be engaged in a helping relationship.

In a review of effective cognitive-behavioural supervision, Milne and James (2000) drew attention to investigations that have a significant cognitive-behavioural methodology underpinning the delivery of supervision and consultancy. However, while this work highlights the potency of close monitoring of the supervisee's work, modelling competence, providing specific instructions, goal setting and providing verbal feedback on supervisee performance, it does not evaluate a particular cognitive-behavioural supervision framework (see Fenell et al 1986, Fleming et al 1996, Parsons & Reid 1995, Parsons et al 1993, Realon et al 1983, Russell & Petrie 1994, Schepis & Reid 1994). None the less, the following discussion illustrates how these important aspects can be incorporated into the delivery of cognitive therapy supervision (Box 5.1).

BOX 5.1	An example of a CT supervision agenda based on Liese and Beck (1997:121)

- Personal update
- Agenda setting
- Link to last supervision session
- Previously supervised cases
- Check on homework task
- Discussion of agenda items
- Assignment of new homework
- Summary and feedback from supervisee

CT supervision is educational in that the supervisor provides information, models skills, incorporates practice and provides positive and corrective feedback. CT supervision may also include review of audiotapes and videotapes of supervisees' work (Temple & Bowers 1998). The supervisor aims to help supervisees apply CT as well as they can and to develop their assessment, conceptualization and treatment skills (Paolo 1998). This framework promotes a collaborative approach and encourages the clinical supervisor and supervisee to work as a team; the supervisee is encouraged to be an active participant, formulate supervision questions and make a major contribution to the agenda for each session and participate in methods which foster learning.

Christine Padesky, widely renowned as a luminary of CT training and supervision, also supports the parallel between treatment and supervision processes (Padesky 1996). However, she differentiates supervision modes from supervision foci. A supervision mode is the means by which supervisee learning and discovery occurs. For example:

- using case discussion,
- role play,
- observation (direct or via audio or video recordings),
- co-therapy,
- provision of relevant educational literature.

Rather than be confined to one mode, it is important for the clinical supervisor to use the broad range suggested by Padesky (1996); observation as an adjunct to discussions based on self-report and the therapist's reactions to the therapeutic process.

Observation as an adjunct to discussions based on self-report

Observation of clinical practice, rather than exclusive use of case discussion, is widely supported in the psychotherapy literature generally, and the cognitive therapy literature specifically. It was Rogers (1942) and Corner (1942) who revolutionized the process of supervision in psychotherapy when they introduced the review of audio recordings of therapy sessions, involving the supervisee and their clients, in the context of CS. The audio recording is still one of the most widely used sources of information for supervisors and supervisees working in the psychotherapy, including cognitive psychotherapy, psychology and counselling, professions (Bernard & Goodyear 1998).

Scaife (2001) pointed out that the use of audio recordings of therapy sessions can be beneficial in supervision and goes as far as to suggest this method may offer particular advantages over other media. Audio recordings provide an opportunity for a detailed review of client–therapist interactions, increase accountability and can enhance therapist empathy. Moreover, they create an opportunity to participate and then observe. Consequently, it is argued that time is made available in CS to slow down the interpersonal processes occurring during the therapeutic endeavour. A detailed exploration of the therapist's perceptions and further consideration of their meanings in light of this reflection can be made available.

Supervisees should be encouraged to listen to the recording and decide what areas they want to review in the supervision session. It is the supervisee who formulates their 'supervision question' (Padesky 2002). This may be influenced by what they want to gain from a particular session, what areas of their clinical practice are causing them concern, skills that they may be developing or aspects of their clinical work of which they are uncertain. Sometimes it will be necessary for the supervisor to consider the entire recording and provide appropriate feedback. This is time-consuming for the supervisor but nevertheless extremely beneficial. Obtaining informed consent from the supervisee's client and ensuring the safe storage of these recordings is paramount.

- After obtaining your patient/client's consent, audiorecord an interaction that occurred in clinical practice. Alternatively, you may wish to do this with one of your clinical supervision sessions.
- On reflection, after having listened to the tape: What did you discover? Did your interactions come across as expected? What aspects are you pleased and satisfied with? Do you think you could you have done things differently? How might you have changed things?

Therapist's reactions to the therapeutic process

According to Padesky (1996), the foci of supervision can be the mastering of new skills, conceptualizing clinical problems or progressing the therapist's understanding of the client–therapist relationship. Many cognitive therapy educationalists now highlight the importance of becoming aware of our own cognitions, emotions and behaviour in our therapeutic work with clients. This can facilitate our understanding of CT methods and processes and can also help us to conceptualize treatment plans for clients. During the supervisory process it will sometimes become apparent to a supervisor that a supervisee may have an underlying assumption about a client, the therapy process or the supervisor which is compromising their application of CT, compromising their self-care and/or influencing the process of therapeutic change in a contradictory way. In this regard, cognitive therapy supervision acknowledges the need to explore therapists' reactions to the therapeutic process.

CT supervision does not aim to provide personal CT for supervisees. The purpose of supervision and subsequent content of discussion in CS differs dramatically from therapy. Instead, this exploration aims to increase awareness of how our own cognitions can influence the therapeutic endeavour and how we can use this as a vehicle to understand the issues that can arise during the process of CT. Of course, uncovering the supervisee's thoughts and feelings about their relationship with clients has, 'the added modelling effect of showing him or her how to work through similar emotions in the client' (Schmidt 1979:282). The following example (Case Study 1) illustrates how the cognitive model of supervision can guide a focus on therapist reactions during CS. In the example which follows, the supervisory relationship had been longstanding and the issues discussed related to the supervision agreement established at the outset of the relationship.

CASE STUDY 1: A worked example of CT supervision

Supervision Foci:
Conceptualization and mastery of cognitive therapy techniques

Supervisory Modes:
Case discussion and review of audio recording of therapy session

This supervision session began with the supervisee claiming 'I don't know what to do next.' The supervisee proceeded to describe a recent therapy session with a client suffering from depression and anxiety following a diagnosis of dementia (early stages — mild). The supervisee had correctly identified the client's 'catastrophic thinking' as influential in her psychological distress. When the client stated 'I can't do anything, I'm useless and incapable,' the supervisee intervened with positive comments about the client's achievements. To the supervisee's surprise, the client agreed but with a rapid downturn in her mood. It was this that stimulated the supervisee's uncertainty in what to do next. During the supervision session, the supervisor attempted to make sense of these interactions using Socratic questioning and review of the audio recording of the therapy session. Socratic questioning involves asking the supervisee questions which they have the knowledge to answer, draw the supervisee's attention to information which may be relevant but outwith their current focus and synthesize this new knowledge to re-evaluate their previous conclusion or construct a new idea. The short excerpt that follows provides an example of the style of the Socratic questioning approach.

Supervisee: She was saying she is useless, incapable and can't do anything. She looked disheartened, avoiding eye contact, speaking quietly. I knew this was just her biased thinking so reminded her of the stuff she had achieved recently. Whilst I was giving her these positives she seemed to sink further ... And I got a bit lost.

Supervisor: Tell me a bit more about that?

Supervisee: She was down already, being hard on herself, I intervened by reminding her of this stuff she had been doing and her mood went down further. And that's what I was trying to avoid, making her more distressed ... I think at that point I felt quite panicky, lost ...

Supervisor: So noticing her low mood, avoiding eye contact with you, speaking quietly, and her stating these negative comments, you thought?

Supervisee: I need to make her feel better, improve her mood, get her out of that dark hole.

Supervisor: And failing to do that would mean?

Supervisee: I wasn't doing my job properly ... I should be able to make her feel better.

Supervisor: What does that sound like?

Supervisee: (Giggling) Yes, I know, it's one of my own beliefs. 'I should be able to make her feel better,' yes that's a particularly strong belief I have.

Supervisor: So part of you was thinking 'I need to make her feel better.' And in that situation, it sounds like that belief contributed towards you feeling panicky, and lost?

Supervisee: Ah huh, that's right. I was trying to make her feel less distressed, but the opposite was happening. I wasn't doing my job.

Supervisor: I'm wondering if that had been around when you'd been met with her thinking she was incapable, useless?

Supervisee: Absolutely, those words felt quite powerful, and I wanted to steer away from them.

Supervisor: So staying with her sense of being incapable, useless would mean?

Supervisee: She'd end up feeling worse, more distressed ... And I was unsure about that.

Supervisor: If you'd stayed with her sense of being incapable, your concern was about making her worse, does that sound right?

Supervisee: Yes that's right.

The supervisee was encouraged to review their conceptualization of this case. Reviewing the audio recording of the therapy session facilitated discussion and subsequent discovery of the supervisee's reasons for affirming the client, that is, his underlying assumptions causing this reaction to the client — he observed her distress when reporting on her experiences resulting from her dementia and didn't want the client's mood to deteriorate and wondered what he would do if she became distressed. The supervisee was able to identify some of his own unhelpful underlying assumptions:

'If I explore her sense of being incapable then I'll make her feel worse'
'I should be able to make my client feel better'
'If my client ends up in more distress then it shows I'm not a good therapist'

Having clarified these principles it was then necessary to evaluate their value in the context of the supervisee's current therapeutic relationship. The supervisor guided the supervisee's awareness of the impact of 'avoiding' the client's distress and not following through the 'meaning making process' in relation to the client's view of being 'useless' and 'incapable'. Through guided discovery the supervisee was able to acknowledge the necessity to explore the client's sense of being 'useless' and 'incapable'. This process helped the supervisee develop his case formulation which subsequently informed his future interventions. More importantly, this stimulated the supervisee to do further work on his own underlying assumptions. He eventually identified the following alternatives:

'If I explore a client's perspective then they will feel better understood'

'If my client becomes distressed then it highlights the significance of what is being discussed'

'If my client becomes upset then I can provide a safe environment for them to express these feelings, I can ask the client for feedback on this aspect of the session and the session generally'

Following some role play demonstrations, the supervisee proceeded to engage with this client and some others guided by these new principles as a behavioural experiment to evaluate their usefulness.

While this psychotherapy-based model has been designed for use by cognitive therapists, it is suggested that the structure and process of this supervisory model might be of value to other healthcare professionals where the concepts of supervisory foci and modes of delivery are equally applicable and where the supervisee seeks an educational focus (Sloan 1999a) and the supervisor aims to guide discovery on the supervisee's therapeutic work. Interested readers wishing a more comprehensive review of CT supervision are referred to Liese and Beck (1997) and Padesky (1996). Table 5.1, from an actual supervision session, outlines the main agenda items within a supervision session (see Box 5.1) but now includes specific examples of questions that a supervisor working in the mental health specialty might ask.

TABLE 5.1 *Helpful questions for supervision in a mental health nursing speciality*

Personal update	How are things with you?
Agenda setting	What items do you want to highlight for our agenda today? What's your supervision question today?
Link to last session	What did you find useful from our last session? Has there been anything from our last session that you've incorporated into your practice? Anything unhelpful from the last session?
Check on homework task from a previously supervised case	You were going to practise incorporating an agenda with some of your clients to explore how helpful/unhelpful that is, how did that go?
Discussion of agenda items	For example, review an audio recording of a recent nurse–patient interaction.
Assignment of new homework	What do you think would be useful for you to work on for next session?
Summary and feedback	What aspects of today's session have been helpful/unhelpful? Is there anything else I can do to help?

Using a CT supervision framework/structure in your own supervision
- Compare and contrast the supervision documentation you are currently using as a supervisee/supervisor in practice with the structure in Box 5.2.
- Why not experiment with or adapt the structure in Box 5.2 for your next clinical supervision session and use this as a discussion item at the end of your session?
- You might now wish to follow this up by obtaining and reading the article by Sloan and colleagues (Sloan et al 2000).

Evidence base for cognitive therapy supervision

Despite a commitment to evidence-based practice in cognitive-behavioural therapy, empirical data on the efficacy of cognitive therapy supervision are minimal. When the cognitive therapy supervision framework is considered with reference to the research literature relating to those characteristics which have been identified as necessary for effective supervision (Balsam & Garber 1970, Rich 1993, Russell & Petrie 1994) it becomes obvious that the cognitive therapy supervision model aligns with much of this evidence: for example, providing the opportunity for the supervisee to observe his or her supervisor's clinical practice, demonstrate and encourage the use of new skills using role play, and providing relevant educational literature (Worthington & Roehlke 1979) providing guidance with treatment and direction with therapeutic interventions (Rabinowitz et al 1986, Worthington 1984) and having the relevant knowledge, clinical skills and teaching ability (Fowler 1995). Another fundamental requirement of effective supervision evident in the cognitive therapy framework is its supportive nature (Fowler 1995, Rabinowitz et al 1986, Sloan 1999b, Worthen & McNeill 1996, Worthington 1984, Worthington & Roehlke 1979).

By using such a highly structured and clinically focused framework for CS the possibility of conducting realistic evaluative research becomes attainable. Adherence to the cognitive therapy supervision process could be evidenced using a modified version of the CT scale (Young & Beck 1980) or the Evaluation of Supervisor form developed by Judith Beck (2005) at the Beck Institute for Cognitive Therapy and Research. More importantly, because the cognitive therapy model remains loyal to the fundamental intention of CS, development of the supervisee's therapeutic competence, its effect on the progression of skills for the supervisee could be evaluated. Perhaps then, the benefit of CS for client well-being could be more readily evidenced.

CLINICAL SUPERVISION GUIDED BY SIX CATEGORY INTERVENTION ANALYSIS

Heron's six category intervention analysis is a conceptual model which was initially developed to progress the understanding of interpersonal relations, and specifically to assist the delivery of interventions within a helping paradigm; hence its consideration in this chapter under psychotherapy-based supervision models. Since 1975 the model has been influential in helping mental health nurses develop a framework for their interactions with patients (Ashmore 1999, Chambers 1990, Hammond 1983). Burnard (1985, 2002) popularized Heron's work for general nursing settings. He suggested that the nurse who develops competence in the six categories of intervention could become an effective helper in a broad range of interpersonal contexts. More recently, six category intervention analysis has been put forward as a suitable model to guide the delivery of CS in nursing (Chambers & Long 1995, Cutcliffe & Epling 1997).

According to Heron (1976), the interpersonal relationship takes place between a practitioner and client. A practitioner is defined as anyone who offers a professional service to a client, so the term refers equally to doctor, psychiatrist, psychotherapist, nurse, lawyer, and teacher, for example. The client is the person who chooses to involve him- or herself in the service that the practitioner is offering, in order to meet a need the client has identified.

The six category system describes six basic kinds of intention a practitioner can have when working with a client. Prescriptive interventions seek to influence and direct the behaviour of the client and include offering advice and making suggestions. To be informative is to offer information or instruction. Heron (1989:38) stated that 'informative interventions seek to impart to the client new knowledge, information and meaning that is relevant to their needs and interests'. Confronting interventions directly challenge the rigid and maladaptive ways that limit the client. A confronting intervention tells an uncomfortable truth 'but does so with love, in order that the client concerned may see it and fully acknowledge it' (Heron 1989:45). Cathartic interventions assist the client to abreact painful emotion, for example, grief, fear and anger. The interventions are pitched at a level of distress which the person is ready to deal with. Heron claimed that cathartic and confronting interventions were those on which participants at his workshops rated themselves weakest. Catalytic interventions include encouraging further self-exploration, self-directed living, learning and problem-solving in the client. Lastly, to be supportive is to validate or confirm the worth of the client's person, qualities, attitudes or actions.

BOX 5.2	*Examples of interventions*

Prescriptive

Supervisee: 'I'm not sure about the motives of client x'

Supervisor: 'I think you should discharge him.... yes just discharge him'

Informative

Supervisee: What's OCD again?

Supervisor: OCD stands for obsessive-compulsive disorder.

Confronting

Supervisee: I'm fed up with this client, he never does any homework tasks I set.

Supervisor: How involved is your client when agreeing homework?

BOX 5.2	*(cont'd)*

Supervisee: I tell him what he has to do between sessions.

Supervisor: And when you do that what happens?

Supervisee: (medium pause) Right, so I shouldn't be telling him what to do.

Supervisor: That method of assigning homework doesn't seem to be working, I'm wondering if that's something you've discussed with this client, his thoughts about your suggestions for homework?

Supervisee: No I've never asked, you're right, I'll write that down and discuss it with him at the next session.

Cathartic

Supervisee: So I've got 70 patients on my list, they all seem so complex, various needs and broad range of problems. I never seem to get any time to think about what I'm doing, I'm too busy for that. So I try and make time but my diary is too full (medium pause, supervisee's eyes fill up with tears).

Supervisor: And thinking about all this stuff just now is upsetting you. I want to help, tell me some more about these pressures.

Catalytic

Supervisee: I don't know what to do, apply for the local course or wait till next year and apply for that one over in the East coast.

Supervisor: Sounds like there might be advantages and disadvantages for both those options?

Supervisee: What would you do?

Supervisor: I'm not sure if my choice would be the right choice for you. How do you feel about thinking some more about each of these options, weighing up the pluses and minuses for each?

Supervisee: Yes, that would be helpful.

Supervisor: Okay, so what are the options …?

Supportive

Supervisee: So I've managed to write out my care plan for this chap.

Supervisor: That is excellent, cause last time you felt a bit stuck and unsure about certain aspects of his experiences … Good for you, I like how you've made reference to some of the relevant research and bullet-pointed your rationale for these interventions. Excellent work.

In addition to describing helpful interventions, the framework also highlights strategies that can be considered degenerate and perverted (Heron 1989). He elaborated:

> To say that an intervention is degenerate, in the sense intended here, is not to say that it is deliberately malicious or perverted (I deal with this type later); but rather that it is misguided, rooted in lack of awareness — lack of experience, of insight, of personal growth, or simply of training.
> Heron, 1989:149

Four degenerate interventions are described: unsolicited, manipulative, compulsive and unskilled. An unsolicited intervention occurs when, without being asked, the practitioner starts to interact in a particular way with the client without any agreement, negotiation or permission, for example, advising that the client do something when this has not been asked for, or offering therapy when this is not appropriate to the task at hand. Manipulative interventions are motivated by the practitioner's self-interest regardless of the interests of the client; the practitioner gets what they want out of the interaction. Heron highlighted that compulsive interventions can be punitive, colluding or evasive and are rooted in the practitioner's unresolved psychological material. Lastly, unskilled interventions result from the practitioner's incompetence in interpersonal skills (Box 5.3).

BOX 5.3	***Examples of unsolicited and unskilled degenerate interventions***

Prescriptive degenerate intervention (unsolicited)

Supervisee: Right, I'm not looking for answers here but I'm not sure about this client. He attends all appointments, takes away the homework I've given him, but never does it. He always looks so guilty for not having done the work and I feel sorry for him so do nothing more … it would be helpful to explore my relationship with this chap.

Supervisor: It's one thing him turning up for appointments and another failing to do the homework … you should discharge him, seriously, you'll get nowhere with him, just discharge him.

Informative degenerate intervention (unskilled)

Supervisee: I've been seeing this chap, suffers from psychosis, first episode, encouraging him to talk about his experiences.

Supervisor: I'm not sure allowing him to talk about his experiences will be that useful, you'll just reinforce his wacky ideas … is he on medication? That's the best thing for these kinds, plenty of medication, stops the delusions.

While degenerate interventions are rooted in lack of awareness, lack of experience, lack of personal growth or a lack of training, perverted interventions are, according to Heron (1989), something darker. Perverted interventions are malicious and intentionally harmful, and, in their execution, the practitioner sets out to do damage to the client. Heron highlighted that such interventions are, in usual circumstances, nothing to do with normal practitioner–client interactions.

The Allitt inquiry (Clothier et al 1994) illustrates an example of perverse interventions at the extreme end of the spectrum. Chambers and Long (1995), Cutcliffe and Epling (1997), Driscoll (2000a), Fowler (1996) and Johns and Butcher (1993) have described a model for CS based on John Heron's (1989) theoretical framework. Descriptions of the six category intervention analysis (Heron 1989) in the context of nurses pursuing a counselling qualification (Chambers & Long 1995, Cutcliffe & Epling 1997), pursuing a degree (Chambers & Long 1995), working in respite care (Johns & Butcher 1993) and working in paediatric nursing (Devitt 1998) have been published. More recently, Sloan (2004) used this framework to undertake secondary analysis of supervisor–supervisee interactions and found that catalytic, informative and supportive interventions were used most frequently; cathartic and confronting interventions were rarely observed during supervision sessions.

Based on the work of John Heron (2001)

- What sorts of intervention do you tend to use most and least in your work with clients/patients?
- What sorts of intervention do you tend to use most and least during your supervision sessions — whether as a supervisee/supervisor (or both)?
- What might be the implications for your patients/clients or in supervision of the above? How possible is it to change your types of intervention? What would need to happen?
- Have there been times when you've intervened in a degenerate fashion?

In the following example of an informative intervention, taken from an audio recording of a supervision session, the clinical supervisor shares some of his own personal experiences (Case Study 2). Prior to conveying this information, Daniel (clinical supervisor) and Claire (supervisee) had been discussing the difficulties Claire was having in keeping up to date with all her paperwork.

CASE STUDY 2: A worked example of supervision using an informative intervention

Daniel: The way I work my documentation Claire and I really can't compare it directly because you've got a far higher caseload, numbers and intensity but I'm covering some visits for Iona just now and I was up at (local village) yesterday afternoon. Now I had my day planned out, and my day was planned out in such a way that I knew that when I had finished my visits at (local village) that I'd be stopping between (local village) and (local village) in a lay-by right, switching the car off, putting the windows down, open my case, getting my notes done and dictating, I think I did about three letters.

Claire: Um.

Daniel: Now, (brief pause) if I hadn't have done that on the lay-by I would have been straight down to the office. I would have come into the office, there would have been messages lying, they would have been this ... So and that has been a practice of mine for years now. So I mean, for example, six years ago or that when I had the (local village) practice, same thing, I would take my notes with me, and on the road back down, into the lay-by, notes all filled in before I came back to the office.

There were many examples of informative interventions observed during Daniel's supervision of Claire. As was found in other case sites, the main source of knowledge shared during CS was experiential and in particular the supervisor's own previous experiences (Sloan 2004, 2006).

In his book: Helping the Client (Heron 2001), John Heron provides readers with a wealth of useful interventions for each of the six categories and anyone interested in this approach is strongly encouraged to consult this text. Indeed, this is a major advantage of this framework. Clinical supervisors have a broad resource of suggestions with which they can experiment. On the other hand, many of these interventions have little or no empirical support and should be used cautiously and only when other, validated methods have been attempted.

SOLUTION-FOCUSED CLINICAL SUPERVISION

Driscoll (2000b) described a supervision framework based on solution-focused therapy (de Shazer 1985). The founders of solution-focused therapy (SFT) claim that the model evolved from clinical practice. De Shazer and colleagues discovered that clients were helped just as effectively by engaging in talk about the future as by talking about their problem-laden past. This approach is guided by the following principles:

- The way of working does not have to be hard or complex.
- Things from the past that have worked but have been forgotten can be reutilized.
- The work is collaborative.
- Responsibility for 'work' lies with the client.

The approach endorses key interventions which include 'encouraging the client to do something different', 'look for exceptions to the problem', and 'notice what you would like to see continue in your life', as well as scaling and asking the miracle question. The primary purpose of scaling is to set client goals, measure progress and establish priorities. The miracle question is usually asked in the first session and aims to identify existing solutions and resources and to clarify the client's goals. The miracle question was devised by de Shazer and normally follows a standard formula:

> Imagine when you go to sleep one night a miracle happens and the problems we've been talking about disappear. As you were asleep, you did not know that a miracle had happened. When you woke up what would be the first signs for you that a miracle had happened?
> de Shazer, 1988

Emphasis is also placed on setting achievable goals and the use of goal-directed questions to promote change. The solution-focused therapist helps the client define the problem so that clear, simple and attainable goals can be generated.

In SFT the therapist tries to clarify with clients what they hope will happen should therapy be successful and may ask:

> What will be the first signs for you that you don't need to continue with therapy?
> O'Connell, 1998:49

The change discourse of SFT includes the elements 'competence talk', 'exception talk', 'context-changing talk' and 'deconstructing the problem'. These elements encourage the therapist to identify and affirm strengths and qualities of the client which can be used in solving the problem. The client's coping mechanisms are acknowledged and endorsed during therapy. Furthermore, the therapist engages with the client in seeking exceptions to the problem, examples of when the problem is not happening. In SFT abstract words such as depression, self-esteem and anxiety are replaced with a detailed description of the client's day-to-day behaviour.

Perhaps the assumptions underpinning solution-focused therapy, as suggested by Driscoll (2000b), are applicable to the CS encounter. Instead of supervision having a problem focus, supervision guided by SFT encourages supervisor and supervisee to explore solutions. Using this psychotherapy-based supervision model, the emphasis is on strengths, resources and exceptions to when problems are encountered. This approach would appear to have considerable benefits for healthcare professionals, particularly when consideration is given to the fact that opportunities to focus on strengths and affirmation of good work are so rare. Similarly, focusing on problems at every opportunity of CS may do little for either the supervisor or supervisee's confidence.

Lowe and Guy (1996) and Edwards and Chen (1999) have written about the SFT-based supervision model and interested readers should follow up on these references. In a recent publication, Lowe and Guy (2002) described six major areas of inquiry which occur in a typical CS session. These are:

- Clarifying hopes and priorities for the session.
- Appreciating competence and change.
- Identifying challenges and resources.
- Contributing ideas and perspectives.
- Discussing future possibilities.
- Reflecting on the session.

For the purposes of this chapter three of these areas will be described: clarifying hopes and possibilities for the session, appreciating competence and change and discussing future possibilities. These have been chosen for further elaboration because of their relevance to other healthcare professionals as they engage in CS. Clarifying hopes and expectations provides a platform from which discussions can develop. Appreciating competence encourages those participating in CS to consider strengths and change implies action following supervision discussions. Finally, discussing future possibilities reinforces the necessity to follow through on ideas which evolve during CS.

In solution-focused frameworks, a session usually begins with clarification of the therapist's hopes and priorities for the meeting. The clinical supervisor may ask:

How would you like to use your session?
How will you know we've done some good work?

Notice the emphasis placed on the generation of supervisee ideas for the session but also how it is the supervisee's views on the benefits of the session that will be used to determine 'good work'.

As mentioned earlier when using other models of CS there is often too much focus on problem talk; strengths, achievements and successes are rarely brought into view. This oversight is addressed during SFT-based supervision when space is made available to appreciate competence and change. In this context the clinical supervisor might ask:

What aspects of your work with this client are you satisfied with?
How would your client describe how you have helped?
How have you developed as a therapist during the past 12 months?

In keeping with its goal-oriented approach and moving things forward to the next area, 'discussing future possibilities' provides an opportunity for supervisor and supervisee to contemplate how their work during the session can impact on the supervisee's clinical work. Essentially this facilitates some connection between the major themes of the discussion and potential future actions. The clinical supervisor may ask:

In relation to what we've discussed, have you any thoughts about what you
    might do in the next session with your client?
If you were working more effectively with this client, what would they notice?

There have been problems in evidencing the benefits of CS and perhaps the problem focus during supervision has contributed to this. When using the SFT-based supervision model, emphasis is given to solutions and actions. Consequently, positive change resulting from CS may be more observable when the SFT approach is adopted.

It has been suggested that what contributes to the effectiveness of CS extends beyond the adoption of a particular framework. Using any one of these approaches to guide CS will not be enough. Recognition has been given to the contribution of the supervisory relationship. The following section provides an overview of the literature pertaining to the supervisory relationship and its influence on effective CS.

EVALUATING THE EFFECTIVENESS OF PSYCHOLOGICAL APPROACHES IN CLINICAL SUPERVISION

According to Russell and Petrie (1994), regardless of the specific theoretical model or the level of the supervisee, a supportive, facilitative supervisory relationship is deemed critical to effective CS; those personal qualities that contribute to creating a nurturing environment are the most essential. Box 5.4 lists some of the personal qualities and characteristics of effective CS, compiled from a variety of sources (see Allan et al 1986, Carifio & Hess 1987, Fowler 1995, Heppner & Roehlke 1984, Loganbill et al 1982, Nelson 1978, Pesut & Williams 1990, Rabinowitz et al 1986, Severinsson 1995, Severinsson & Hallberg 1996, Sloan 1999, Worthington 1984).

BOX 5.4	*List of personal qualities and characteristics of effective CS*

Sense of humour

Integrity

Trustworthy

Honest

Competent

Understanding

Sensitive

Tactful

Supportive

Credible

Genuine

Tolerant

Encouraging

Clarifies expectations

Maintains consistent and appropriate boundaries

Has knowledge of theory and current research

Is accessible and available

Provides constructive criticism and positive feedback

Creates a relaxed learning environment

Is aware of and accepts own limitations and strengths

Works collaboratively

Teaches practical skills

Teaches case conceptualization

While lists of qualities and characteristics can be generated for both effective and ineffective CS, little is known about what kind of supervision is going to be effective with a particular supervisee in any given situation. Clinical supervisor and supervisee need to work together to determine what specific qualities, behaviours, methods and techniques are going to be most effective for their particular circumstances and supervision agreement (see Chapter 4 for further discussion). Empirical research is relatively sparse for the CS of qualified practitioners. A lot of work has been undertaken with beginning supervisees in academic settings but little is known about what supervisory interventions are needed to encourage growth to the higher stages of therapeutic competence.

A key aspect of the psychological approaches described in this chapter is the description they provide regarding their essential components. As mentioned earlier, Heron's framework provides a valuable resource of helpful ways of interacting. What are required now are research studies investigating the particular value of the different sorts of interventions in each of the six categories for the purpose of CS. It would also be useful to explore the merits of each of the six categories and the specific contexts within which they are delivered.

The SFT model of CS encourages us to consider solutions rather than get bogged down by the problems inherent in clinical practice. This framework emphasizes the requirement for change, which when attempting to measure the effectiveness of CS, would be an important consideration.

In the CT model of CS, when using specific modes of delivery and foci, the content remains focused on developing the supervisee's therapeutic competence. Consequently, this structure guides discovery of the therapist's or helper's mission — the provision of effective therapeutic/helpful interactions. This would be an important focus for future CS research. Furthermore, in this framework a distinction is made between supervision modes and foci. Future research could compare the effectiveness of the case discussion with reviewing audio recordings of interactions in developing supervisee skills.

CONCLUSION

It has been acknowledged that CS has major benefits for nurses and other healthcare professionals. None the less, as argued elsewhere (Sloan & Watson 2001), some of these expectations may distract from other equally important outcomes. In describing some of the psychotherapy-based supervision models, it is intended that this chapter provides some guidance on how CS can have a client focus, the therapeutic alliance between supervisee and their clients, the foundation upon which therapeutic interventions can be delivered.

There are significant barriers to having such a specific focus for CS. CS is an expensive, time-consuming activity, which does take practitioners away from direct clinical work. Consequently, major stakeholders want to gain as much as possible from CS. Not surprisingly, CS often ends up having a broad scope. But there are other concerns. CS is often used to discuss management issues and if it was used for the sole purpose as described in this chapter, other opportunities for managerial supervision would have to be made available. Similarly, CS is often understood as a supportive resource to improve the emotional wellbeing of the supervisee. If practitioners engage in CS to focus on client-related concerns other opportunities of support and evidence-based stress-relieving interventions will be required.

Engaging in CS with the intention of enhancing client care may provide opportunities for more realistic outcome research. In this regard, future research could investigate the therapeutic work of healthcare professionals, mental health nurses or occupational therapists as explored during CS, for example. Furthermore, the contribution of CS to this therapeutic work could be investigated. A useful study might be to explore how reviewing audio recordings of practitioner–patient interactions during CS affects subsequent interactions. Similarly, what are the benefits of reviewing audio recordings of practitioner–patient interactions over the case discussion method?

Future research should also consider the supervisory relationship and its impact on the outcomes from CS. More research investigating effective CS for qualified and experienced practitioners is certainly required. Furthermore, we need to explore the types and styles of supervisor–supervisee interactions which contribute to particular outcomes of CS. Do prescriptive interventions from the clinical supervisor lead to knowledge acquisition in the supervisee or do they undermine self-confidence?

It is hoped that readers' interest in these psychological approaches will be stimulated, that they follow up with further reading and experimentation. With this in mind, I would encourage interested readers to locate a supervisor, who has received psychotherapy and supervision training and is able to guide supervision using a psychological framework, and experience further discoveries for yourself. I have every confidence that your engagement in CS will be enhanced as a consequence.

On reflection ... chapter summary

- The use of psychological approaches in CS provides an opportunity for the supervisee to consider their contribution to the therapeutic/helping relationship.
- CT supervision endorses interventions which are considered to be effective.
- CT supervision encourages the use of a variety of modes and foci; these emphasize progression of the supervisee's therapeutic competence.
- Heron's framework guides the supervisor in six categories of intervening, that is, prescriptive, informative, confronting, cathartic, catalytic and supportive interventions.
- Degenerative or unhelpful ways of intervening are also described in Heron's framework.
- A key attribute of SFT is its focus on solutions.

REFERENCES

Allan G J, Szollos S J, Williams B E 1986 Doctoral students' comparative evaluations of best and worst psychotherapy supervision. Professional Psychology: Research and Practice 17(7):91–99

Ashmore R 1999 Heron's intervention framework: an introduction and critique. Mental Health Nursing 19(1):24–27

Balsam A, Garber N 1970 Characteristics of psychotherapy supervision. Journal of Medical Education 45(10):789–797

Beck J 2005 Evaluation of supervisors form (revised version). Beck Institute of Cognitive Therapy and Research. Bala Cynwyd, PA

Bernard J M, Goodyear R K 1998 Fundamentals of clinical supervision. Allyn and Bacon, London

Burnard P 1985 Learning human skills: a guide for nurses. Heinemann, London

Burnard P 2002 Learning human skills: an experiential and reflective guide for nurses and healthcare professionals. 4th edn. Butterworth Heinemann, Oxford

Carifio M S, Hess A K 1987 Who is the ideal supervisor? Professional Psychology: Research and Practice 18(3):244–250

Chambers M 1990 Psychiatric and mental health nursing: learning in the clinical environment. In: Reynolds W, Cormack D (eds) Psychiatric and mental health nursing: theory and practice. Chapman and Hall, London, p 396–433

Chambers M, Long A 1995 Supportive clinical supervision: a crucible for personal and professional change. Journal of Psychiatric and Mental Health Nursing 2(5):311–316

Clothier C, MacDonald C A, Shaw D A 1994 The Allitt inquiry: independent inquiry relating to the deaths and injuries on the children's ward at Grantham and Kesteven General Hospital during the period February to April 1991. HMSO, London

Corner B J 1942 Studies in phonographic recordings of verbal material. 1: the use of phonographic recordings in counselling practice and research. Journal of Consulting Psychology 6(1):105–113

Cutcliffe J R, Epling M 1997 An exploration of the use of John Heron's confronting interventions in clinical supervision: Case studies from practice. Psychiatric Care 4(4):174–180

de Shazer S 1985 Keys to solutions in brief therapy. Norton, New York

de Shazer S 1988 Clues: investigating solutions in brief therapy. Norton, New York

Devitt P 1998 A grounded theory investigation into the nature of the supervisory relationship and the labour of supervision through the eyes of the supervisor. Department of Nursing, University of Manchester, Manchester

Doehrmann M J 1976 Parallel processes in supervision and psychotherapy. Bulletin of the Menninger Clinic 40(1):3–104

Driscoll J 2000a Practising clinical supervision: a reflective approach. Bailliere Tindall, London

Driscoll J 2000b Clinical supervision: a radical approach. Mental Health Practice 3(8):8–10

Edwards J K, Chen M 1999 Strength-based supervision: Frameworks, current practice, and future directions. Family Journal: Counselling and Therapy for Couples and Families 17(6):349–357

Faugier J, Butterworth T 1994 Clinical supervision: a position paper. University of Manchester, Manchester

Fenell D L, Hovestadt A J, Harvey S J 1986 A comparison of delayed feedback and live supervision models of marriage and family therapist clinical training. Journal of Marital and Family Therapy 12:181–186

Fleming R K, Oliver J R, Bolton D M 1996 Training supervisors to train staff. Journal of Organizational Behaviour and Management 16(1):3–25

Fowler J 1995 Nurses' perceptions of the elements of good supervision. Nursing Times 91(22):33–37

Fowler J 1996 Clinical supervision: what do you do after you say hello? British Journal of Nursing 5(6):382–385

Hammond J 1983 A clutch of concepts. Nursing Mirror 156(19):34–35

Hawkins P, Shohet R 2000 Supervision in the helping professions. 2nd edn. Open University, Milton Keynes

Heppner P P, Roehlke H J 1984 Differences among supervisees at different levels of training: implications for a development model of supervision. Journal of Counselling Psychology 31(1):76–90

Heron J 1976 A six category intervention analysis. British Journal of Guidance and Counselling 4(2):143–155

Heron J 1989 Six category intervention analysis. University of Surrey. Human Potential Resource Group, Guildford

Heron J 2001 Helping the client: a creative practical guide. 5th edn. Sage, London

Holloway E L, Neufeldt S A 1995 Supervision: its contribution to treatment efficacy. Journal of Consulting and Clinical Psychology 63(2):207–213

Howard F M 1997 Supervision. In: Love H, Whittaker W (eds) Practice issues for clinical and applied psychologists in New Zealand. The New Zealand Psychological Society, Wellington, p 340–358

Johns C, Butcher K 1993 Learning through supervision: a case study of respite care. Journal of Clinical Nursing 2(2):89–93

Kilminster S M, Jolly B C 2000 Effective supervision in clinical practice settings: a literature review. Medical Education 34(10):827–840

Liese B S, Beck J S 1997 Cognitive therapy supervision. In: Watkins C E (ed) Handbook of psychotherapy supervision. Wiley, New York, p 114–133

Loganbill C, Hardy E, Delworth V 1982 Supervision: a conceptual model. Counselling Psychology 10(1):3–42

Lowe R, Guy G 1996 A reflecting team format for solution-oriented supervision: Practical guidelines and theoretical distinctions. Journal of Systemic Therapies 15(1):26–45

Lowe R, Guy G 2002 Solution-oriented inquiry for ongoing supervision: expanding the horizon of change. In: McMahon M, Patton W (eds) Supervision in the helping professions: a practical approach. Pearson Education Australia, NSW, p 143–156

Milne D, James I 2000 A systematic review of effective cognitive-behavioural supervision. British Journal of Clinical Psychology 39(2):111–127

Nelson G L 1978 Psychotherapy supervision from the trainee's point of view: a survey of preferences. Professional Psychology 9(4):539–550

Newman C F 1998 Therapeutic and supervisory relationships in cognitive-behavioural therapies: similarities and differences. Journal of Cognitive Psychotherapy: An International Quarterly 12(2):95–108

O'Connell B 1998 Solution-focused therapy. Sage, London

Padesky C 1996 Developing cognitive therapist competency: teaching and supervision models. In: Salkovskis P M (ed) Frontiers of cognitive therapy. The Guilford Press, London, p 266–292

Padesky C 2002 Cognitive therapy supervision: principles and practice. Centre of Cognitive Therapy, California

Paolo S B 1998 Receiving supervision in cognitive therapy: a personal account. Journal of Cognitive Psychotherapy: An International Quarterly 12(2):154–162

Parsons M B, Reid D H 1995 Training residential supervisors to provide feedback for maintaining staff teaching skills with people who have severe disabilities. Journal of Applied Behaviour Analysis 28:317–322

Parsons M B, Reid D H, Green C W 1993 Preparing direct service staff to teach people with severe disabilities: A comprehensive evaluation of an effective and acceptable training programme. Behavioural Residential Treatment 8:163–185

Pesut D J, Williams C A 1990 The nature of clinical supervision in psychiatric nursing: A survey of clinical specialists. Archives of Psychiatric Nursing 4(3):188–194

Proctor B 1987 Supervision: a co-operative exercise in accountability. In: Marken M, Payne M (eds) Enabling and ensuring: supervision in practice. National Youth Bureau and the Council for Education and Training in Youth and Community Work, Leicester, p 21–34

Rabinowitz F E, Heppner P P, Roehlke H J 1986 Descriptive study of process and outcome variables of supervision over time. Journal of Counselling Psychology 33(3):292–300

Realon R E, Lewallan J D, Wheelan A J 1983 Verbal feedback vs verbal feedback plus praise: the effects on direct care staff's training behaviours. Mental Retardation 21:209–212

Rich P 1993 The form, function, and content of clinical supervision. Clinical Supervisor 11(1):137–178

Rogers C R 1942 The use of electrically recorded interviews in improving psychotherapeutic techniques. American Journal of Orthopsychiatry 12:429–434

Russell R K, Petrie T 1994 Issues in training effective supervisors. Applied Preventive Psychology 3(1):27–42

Safran J, Segal Z 1996 Interpersonal process in cognitive therapy. Jason Aronson, London

Scaife J 2001 Supervision in the mental health professions: a practitioner's guide. Brunner-Routledge, East Sussex

Schepis M M, Reid D H 1994 Training direct service staff in congregate settings to interact with people with severe disabilities: a quick, effective and acceptable programme. Behavioural Interventions 9(1):13–26

Schmidt J P 1979 Psychotherapy supervision: a cognitive-behavioural model. Professional Psychology 10(3):278–284

Severinsson E I 1995 The phenomenon of clinical supervision in psychiatric healthcare. Journal of Psychiatric and Mental Health Nursing 2(5):301–309

Severinsson E I, Hallberg I R 1996 Clinical supervisors' views of their leadership role in the clinical supervision process within nursing care. Journal of Advanced Nursing 24(1):151–161

Sloan G 1999a Good characteristics of a clinical supervisor: a community mental health nurse perspective. Journal of Advanced Nursing 30(3):713–722

Sloan G 1999b The therapeutic relationship in cognitive-behavioural therapy. British Journal of Community Nursing 4(2):58–64

Sloan G 2004 An illuminative evaluation of clinical supervision in mental health nursing. Unpublished PhD Thesis. Department of Nursing and Community Health, Glasgow Caledonian University, Glasgow

Sloan G 2006 Clinical supervision in mental health nursing. Wiley, London

Sloan G, Watson H 2001 Illuminative evaluation: evaluating clinical supervision on its performance rather than the applause. Journal of Advanced Nursing 35(5):664–673

Sloan G, White C, Coit F 2000 Cognitive therapy supervision as a framework for clinical supervision in nursing: using structure to guide discovery. Journal of Advanced Nursing 32(3):515–524

Temple S, Bowers W A 1998 Supervising cognitive therapists from diverse fields. Journal of Cognitive Psychotherapy: An International Quarterly 12(2):139–151

Todd G, Freshwater D 1999 Reflective practice and guided discovery: clinical supervision. British Journal of Nursing 8(20):1383–1389

Van Ooijen E 2000 Clinical supervision: a practical guide. Churchill Livingstone, London

Watkins C E 1990 The separation – individuation process in psychotherapy supervision. Psychotherapy 27(2):202–209

Worthen V, McNeill B W 1996 A phenomenological investigation of 'good' supervision events. Journal of Counselling Psychology 43(1):25–34

Worthington E L 1984 Empirical investigation of supervision of counsellors as they gain experience. Journal of Counselling Psychology 31(1):63–75

Worthington E L, Roehlke H J 1979 Effective supervision as perceived by beginning counsellors-in-training. Journal of Counselling Psychology 26(1):64–73

Yegdich T 1996 Borne to be free: Enduring the unthought known in supervision and therapy. Paper presented at the Rozelle Annual Winter Symposium, July, Sydney, Australia

Yegdich T 1999 Lost in a crucible of supportive clinical supervision: supervision is not therapy. Journal of Advanced Nursing 29(5):1265–1275

Young J, Beck A T 1980 Cognitive therapy scale: rating manual. Unpublished manuscript, University of Pennsylvania, Philadelphia

6

Exploring the potential of professional coaching for the growth of clinical supervision in practice

John Driscoll and Gerard O'Donovan

INTRODUCTION

In this chapter we will examine what coaching is and consider whether some of the core skills used in 'coaching a client' might also have some resonance with what clinical supervisors are trying to achieve in 'supervising a supervisee'. Just as important as what is trying to be achieved in coaching or clinical supervision are the roles of the 'client' and 'supervisee' in the two processes and the nature of the relationship itself. Much of the thinking behind this chapter is borne out of (the first author) John's continuing developmental journey towards becoming an 'accredited coach' and being a recipient of the coaching process. Part of the agreement made with Rachel (John's coach) has been for him to personally experience coaching by utilizing it as a form of clinical supervision. This has enabled him, with the help of Gerard (the second author), to reflect on the potential of coaching practices in clinical supervision situations, while acting as a clinical supervisor in selected UK healthcare settings.

In over a decade of the emergence of clinical supervision in UK healthcare there is some general agreement that the term 'supervision' is not an accurate description of the intentions behind the process and this, in John's view, continues to act as a barrier in getting started in practice. The development of coaching is an unexplored frontier for clinical supervision and its application to the healthcare practice environment.

At the risk of 'muddying the water' (a response a respected academic colleague of John's made to the notion of introducing elements of coaching into clinical supervision) we suggest that coaching, in particular development coaching, has much to offer the clinical supervision encounter, particularly for senior staff supervisees (in terms of conversational structure, being more demonstrable in terms of outcomes, less 'problem' orientated and being a more equal relationship).

For health professionals the term 'development coaching' might more accurately be applied to senior and experienced healthcare staff, reserving the term clinical 'supervision' for more individualized and performance related activities with more junior staff. If this premise is accepted, the implications are enormous in healthcare in terms of developing coaches as well as supervisors and rethinking what already happens in clinical supervision. On the other hand, existing professional coaches, who undergo long training programmes to become accredited, might feel their role is being usurped by healthcare supervisors.

Our view is that both coaching and nursing as professions have an established history of 'borrowing' knowledge from other related disciplines to generally inform their practices, and that the knowledge base of professional coaching, with its emphasis on developing potential and enhancing work performance, has much to offer the development of clinical supervision activities.

Although the chapter is not a broad examination of coaching as a profession *per se*, it seems sensible to question what happens in 'coaching' and analyse the different interventions that might be suitable for use in the clinical supervision encounter. Different types of coaching and a popular coaching framework are outlined, in order to help make some tentative comparisons between the skills used in coaching and clinical supervision. For those of you already engaged in the process of clinical supervision (as a supervisor, supervisee, or supporting the initiative as a healthcare manager) we offer a challenge: consider experimenting with a coaching framework as a potential structure for one of your clinical supervision sessions.

THE LANDSCAPE OF PROFESSIONAL COACHING AS A CLINICAL SUPERVISION CONTINUUM

When one thinks of the term 'coaching', competitive sports and winning are brought to mind (Kinlaw 1997:21, Peltier 2001:170, Starr 2003:5). For instance, how many times do you recall successful sportsmen and women, when they are interviewed shortly after an achievement, making direct references to their coaches as being instrumental to their success? Kelly Holmes, the UK double gold medallist in sprinting, was a perfect example (I am writing this during the 2004 Olympics in Athens).

A coaching model often used in competitive sports is the 'coach' as 'expert' or 'personal trainer'. For example, in golf this might be helping a player towards winning a major tournament or simply remedying aspects of a player's game (such as altering the grip used or perfecting the swing of the club). In the UK, as elsewhere in the world, successful sports team coaches are able to capture a nation's imagination and can even reach legendary status — the late Sir Alf Ramsey (England football World Cup winning coach in 1966) and Sir Clive Woodward (England rugby World Cup winning coach in 2003) to name only two. The reason for this acclaim is simple — successful results.

Effective coaching is not confined to competitive sports; it is evident in other areas that demand high performances. For instance, individualized coaching can enhance the performance of an opera singer and maximize the potential of musicians and others in the performing arts. You can probably think of many other examples in which coaching is cited as improving the abilities or the performance of individuals. Coaching a team, or an individual, to maximize their potential is likely to be based on some of the following attributes of the coach:

- An expert (or having a significant area of expertise).
- A close observer who offers 'live' feedback on technique(s).
- A motivator towards winning ways.
- A setter of ever-increasing levels of performance and endurance.
- A person who is willing to be unpopular when necessary.
- A person who develops a sense of self-belief at 'being the best' or striving toward 'the best they can be'.
- A person who gives time and commitment and expects the same from those being coached.

If as a starting point we agree in principle that coaching (and in particular competitive coaching) is concerned with nurturing potential, maximizing individual or team performance and, most importantly, getting results, it is not surprising that coaching techniques and processes have been applied to the business and industrial sectors. However, Kinlaw (1997:21) points out that a major difference between personal and professional development coaching and sports coaching is that competitive performances often last for a set given period and players only need to be at their best for a defined time span. In contrast, the work of businesses continues unceasingly (unless discontinued) with the consequence that employees are expected to be 'doing their best all of the time' and professional coaching in this situation is a much more complex activity to define.

Although professional coaching might be a new term for many of you, the idea of having a periodic one-to-one conversation with someone (usually a manager) at work about development needs has been around for decades. Jarvis (2004:8) asserts that such conversations are largely based on 'knowing what you need to change' and this is very different from actually helping to bring about those changes in a person's lifestyle or work habits (which is the remit of professional coaching). The rapid expansion of professional coaching is due to a number of changes in the work environment (Box 6.1).

BOX 6.1	*Key factors leading to the expansion of professional coaching in the workplace*
	- Keeping pace and learning to adapt to increasing amounts of change
	- Flatter organizational structures and broader management roles requiring individualized support
	- Learning being considered lifelong and needing to take account of individual learning styles
	- Targeted and responsive approaches to individual development

BOX 6.1	(cont'd)

- **The cost of poor performers to the organization**
  - Formalized support for those at the top who are often isolated or a significant distance from employees
  - Employees having to take individual responsibility as they can no longer rely on employers to provide all their career development

- **The cost-effectiveness of work-based learning schemes as opposed to just the training room of an educational provider**
  - Keeping up the momentum and support with published personal and professional development plans
  - Flexible and individually tailored learning to increase an employee's performance

Adapted from Jarvis (2004:6)

This has in turn led to the surfacing of different areas of coaching expertise, such as personal life coaching, executive coaching and corporate coaching to name but a few. More detailed accounts of the different types of coaching can be found in Hadikin (2004:15), Jarvis (2004:24) and Jay (2001). Interestingly, the term 'clinical supervision' was cited in the early 1980s as a method of coaching teachers for higher performance and transforming the work culture in North American schools (Anderson & Snyder 1993:32). Despite such diversity, all professional coaching maintains that the development of relationships between people and the conversations that take place will have different emphases, depending on the context and the needs of the people being coached.

Downey's (1999:15) broad definition of coaching might also be a definition of individualized clinical supervision in practice:

> Coaching (clinical supervision) is the art of facilitating the performance, learning and development of another.

West and Milan (2001) identify three specific types of coaching for leadership which help to further illustrate the different emphases in the coaching relationship:

- Skills coaching.
- Performance coaching.
- Development coaching.

Skills coaching relates to developing specific skills and abilities in the client for which the coaching parameters and expected outcomes are clearly defined from the beginning, e.g. improving presentation skills at meetings or delivering a conference paper. The relationship may involve directly instructing the client or offering advice and in essence 'training' the client. What distinguishes skills coaching from training is that it is delivered on a one-to-one basis rather than in a large group situation. Skills coaching is a highly individualized and intensive relationship, focusing on the specific learning needs of the client, and is usually short term.

(Although similar to mentoring, skills coaching is different; a mentor either implicitly or explicitly assesses a person's individual level of skill against organizational or professional competencies. A mentor relationship typically involves an experienced senior staff member and a junior staff member. The senior staff member is recruited from within the organization and is expected to directly influence the way the more junior member of staff works; in other words, this is an apprentice–master relationship.)

Performance coaching is wider in scope than skills coaching and intends to enhance a client's general performance in their role at work (by helping the development of particular behaviours or by raising their awareness of behaviours that limit performance). In this respect there is an expectation that coaching will produce results in a client's performance. More often than not the client's role and expected behaviours are defined by the organization as performance objectives or job descriptors. When these objectives are not met, or the client is underperforming, referral for either internal (manager as coach) or external coaching may be necessary.

Thorpe and Clifford (2003:34) not only emphasize the improvement of skills and performance as expected coaching outcomes for the client but also introduce the concept of reflective learning as an important aspect of the process. They define coaching as:

> … the process of helping someone enhance or improve their performance through reflection on how they apply a specific skill and/or knowledge.

Their definition, aimed specifically at the coaching role of a trainer and manager in the workplace, states that the process of coaching facilitates reflection on established sets of competencies or preferred behaviours.

It is interesting to note that the objectives in both skills and performance coaching are clearly defined in the shorter term (over one year) in which results or outcomes can be followed up by the organization in the form of an annual appraisal or personal development review.

Development coaching is usually considered a longer-term investment on the parts of both the organization and the individual, for instance 12 to 18 months (but can last longer), and is a more evolving process than the specific task of skills or performance coaching. (Clinical supervision and development coaching are offered to senior or qualified practitioners and are highly individualized.)

The process begins by initially identifying the agenda and development goals, but more often than not the agenda alters depending on the changing circumstances and complexities of the client's or supervisee's world (West & Milan 2001:10). For instance, in John's development coaching, in which his agenda was to discuss the progress of a large clinical supervision project in prison healthcare, the session changed into ways of valuing what he did and putting a price on services that he offered. In turn this led to a complete re-think on managing his business finances which subconsciously he had been having concerns about.

Timothy Gallwey, a former tennis coach and a major influence on the origins of developmental coaching, based his Inner Game thesis (Gallwey 2000) on the realization that a person's peak performance is often marred by their own 'self-interference'. For example, the self-doubt and fear of failure that interferes with appreciating an individual's potential, let alone peak performance, is not able to be reached.

Based on Gallwey's (2000) Inner Game thesis, how many work colleagues can you think of who are generally more capable than their current performance suggests and in what ways might 'self-interference' manifest itself?

Can you think of either a personal or professional example of how 'self-interference' might be a factor in reducing your own potential or performance?

Gallwey (2000:177) suggests that unlocking a client's potential is not so much a process of adding by the development coach (e.g. new skills or behaviours) but subtracting, or having the client unlearn, whatever is getting in the way of the client reaching that potential. In this respect, the task of the development coach is about facilitating the client's learning or, to be more precise, enabling the client to 'un-learn'. Somers (2002:6) refers to this as 'drawing the client out' rather than 'putting in' and helping to draw on the huge reserves of talent and potential laying dormant in the client.

A key element of development coaching places the client as the main problem solver through gaining an increased sense of self-awareness during reflection on their personal or professional performance and would seem to have distinct parallels to a reflective approach in clinical supervision (previously discussed in Chapter 2).

All three types of coaching outlined (skills, performance or development) present two basic coaching models that can be broadly categorized as either being directive in nature ('showing and telling') or non-directive (the client retains more control in the learning process). Whatever type of coaching is used, all coaching remains outcomes-orientated or performance-focused and is a highly individualized and person-centred endeavour. The two extremes of directive or non-directive coaching activities can be seen as being on a coaching continuum depending on the client's experience and needs and has many similarities with the supervision continuum that already exists in UK healthcare. An adapted coaching/supervision continuum is outlined in Box 6.2 based on the original work of West and Milan (2001:3).

Consider the coaching continuum and the different types of coaching with the healthcare supervision continuum in Box 6.2.
■ Where do you consider yourself to be on the supervision continuum as a healthcare practitioner today?
■ In what ways might the terms skills, performance or development coaching best describe what is currently happening in your own clinical supervision?

In reality there is likely to be some overlap between the three types of coaching or supervision in practice. Most healthcare professionals have undergone lengthy training in which the work of the unqualified practitioner is duly assessed and supervised by a range of more senior qualified practitioners, mentors or trainers. But once qualified, immediate additional skills are then required by a practitioner in making the transition from unqualified to qualified professional. Clinical supervision for the newly qualified junior healthcare professional will initially need to be advisory and directive (e.g. mentoring and preceptoring), focusing on the specific skills of practice. As healthcare practitioners become more experienced and assume more senior roles, they will move towards the right of the coaching-supervision continuum. At this end of

BOX 6.2	An adapted continuum of coaching (Milan & West 2001:3) and its relationship to clinical supervision in UK healthcare (in italics)

SKILLS COACHING   **PERFORMANCE COACHING**   **DEVELOPMENT COACHING**

SUPERVISED PRACTICE AND LEARNING   **ORGANIZATIONAL SUPERVISION**   **SUPPORTIVE SUPERVISION**

TRAINING ⟵⟶ **DEVELOPMENT**

Coaching objectives: finite/concrete	Coaching objectives: complex/emergent
Implied coaching style: directive	Implied coaching style: non-directive
Duration: short term	Duration: long term
Supervision objectives: assessing practitioner safety and competence	Supervision objectives: complex/emergent
Implied supervision style: directive	Implied supervision style: non-directive
Duration: short term	Duration: long term (lifelong learning) and part of a practitioner's continuing professional development (CPD)

the continuum, roles at work become more complex or ambiguous, requiring the less directive skills of development coaching or developmental supervision.

Perhaps junior staff may be considered to be under *clinical supervision* when they are specifically learning skills and/or working to a minimum performance, whereas more senior practitioners may be considered to be either under *developmental supervision* or receiving *development coaching* when they are engaged in continuing professional development (CPD), at which time they will require less direction and more guided reflection.

This gives rise to the question: In what ways might directive or non-directive supervision be a help or a hindrance in clinical practice?

John's personal reflections from his own coaching/supervision with Rachel:

In reality, I would suggest that we all probably have a tendency towards being either directive or less directive depending on our client's or supervisee's needs, which are complex. In my past professional situations, having been a senior practitioner in intensive care and a teacher in a university, I have often been looked upon as an 'expert' with the expectation that I be directive and guide. (In some cases, being directive to others has been life-saving in the clinical situation.)

In contrast, now working as a full-time externally employed change agent and as a freelance consultant, I intend my role to be much less of an 'expert' and directive and more facilitative in nature. As this has not come naturally for me, I am currently 'un'learning this in my own coaching/supervision. I have become much more consciously aware of my old tendencies towards retaining a degree of power and control through having some specific knowledge. My client's expectations are actively wanting me to remain as 'expert', provide answers and at the same time pay me for doing so. The contradiction is that I view my 'expert-ness' at its worst as being potentially counter-productive in fostering a sense of dependency on my services and one which will not be sustained after my contract expires, and at best, not really being facilitative at all. In other words, my being less directive will increase the ownership and subsequent autonomy to act of those that employ my services.

COMPARING CORE DEVELOPMENT COACHING SKILLS TO CLINICAL SUPERVISION

The International Coach Federation (ICF) is a professional organization for coaches based in the USA. Although not an officially recognized regulatory body it does offer some minimum standards and ethical guidelines for coaches and accredits the quality of coaching training programmes. The ICF (2006a) describes the 'what' and 'how' of professional coaching as follows:

> Professional Coaching is an ongoing professional relationship that helps people produce extraordinary results in their lives, careers, businesses or organizations. Through the process of coaching, clients deepen their learning, improve their performance, and enhance their quality of life.

This definition explains what is expected of a coach and is helpful in reflecting on aspects of development coaching that might be useful in the clinical supervision situation. The ICF's notions of professional partnership, goal setting, getting results and relevancy in the one-to-one or group situation aligns with the principles and ideas underpinning clinical supervision.

As part of the standardization of a professional coach's work the ICF (2006b) identifies four key clusters and 11 associated core competencies that are individually examined before a coach can become an accredited member or professional coach (Box 6.3).

| BOX 6.3 | *The four clusters of coaching (ICF 2006b) and 11 associated core competencies* |

Setting the foundation

1) *Meeting ethical guidelines and professional standards* — Understanding of coaching ethics and standards and ability to apply them appropriately in all coaching situations

2) *Establishing the coaching agreement* — Ability to understand what is required in the specific coaching interaction and to come to agreement with the prospective and new client about the coaching process and relationship

Co-creating the relationship

3) *Establishing trust and intimacy with the client* — Ability to create a safe, supportive environment that produces ongoing mutual respect and trust

BOX 6.3	*(cont'd)*

4) *Coaching presence* — Ability to be fully conscious and create spontaneous relationship with the client, employing a style that is open, flexible and confident

Communicating effectively

5) *Active listening* — Ability to focus completely on what the client is saying and is not saying, to understand the meaning of what is said in the context of the client's desires and to support self-expression

6) *Powerful questioning* — Ability to ask questions that reveal the information needed for maximum benefit to the coaching relationship and the client

7) *Direct communication* — Ability to communicate effectively during coaching sessions, and to use language that has the greatest positive impact on the client

Facilitating learning and results

8) *Creating awareness* — Ability to integrate and accurately evaluate multiple sources of information, and to make interpretations that help the client to gain awareness and therby achieve agreed-upon results

9) *Designing actions* — Ability to create with the client opportunities for ongoing learning, during coaching and in work/life situations, and for taking new actions that will most effectively lead to agreed-upon results

10) *Planning and goal setting* — Ability to develop and maintain an effective coaching plan with the client

11) *Managing progress and accountability* — Ability to hold attention on what is important for the client, and to leave responsibility with the client to take action

Another body, the European Coaching Institute (along with other organizations), promotes an industry standard for coaching practices for both individual coaches and training providers (ECI 2006a). There are also published professional Codes of Ethics (EMCC 2004a, ICF 2006a) and Guidelines on Supervision for coaches (Association for Coaching 2005, EMCC 2004b) which demonstrate the effort to continually improve the coaching industry and protect clients.

Taking each of the descriptors of the 11 core competencies of coaching in Box 6.3:
a) Individually rate what you consider to be the appropriateness (or not) of each core competence for use in your clinical supervision situation, i.e. Very Important, Important, Not Important. What is the rationale for the choices you made?
b) For those competencies you rated as Very Important or Important, download the behavioural descriptors from the ICF website and personally rate your current coaching abilities in clinical supervision. What might be the implications for you with this exercise?
c) How useful might each of the 11 core competencies of coaching be in helping to set minimum clinical supervisor behaviours?

The four clusters may offer a useful content for any clinical supervisor training programme and the 11 core competencies a useful discussion point for the future evaluation and perhaps even regulation of clinical supervisor skills. Major difficulties facing existing clinical supervisors in UK healthcare practice is that there is an absence of literature on the subject and virtually no agreement on what the core competencies of a clinical supervisor are in practice. Training courses vary in length and content and in many cases, having undergone a course, clinical supervisors are not required to update or review their knowledge and skills whatever these might be. The current lack of regulation and minimum standards in healthcare clinical supervision therefore leaves the 'doing' of effective clinical supervision to individual interpretation and preference. While it might be argued that adopting a less prescriptive stance for clinical supervision is its strength, there remain unanswered ethical questions about the effects of this on supervisees and what is happening within clinical supervision in organizations.

Using the four clusters of coaching as headings, a number of differences emerge when comparing coaching to clinical supervision (Table 6.1).

TABLE 6.1 *Some key differences between coaching and clinical supervision using the four key clusters of a coach's competence (ICF 2006b)*

	Coaching	Clinical Supervision
Setting the foundation	Incremental levels of coach training based on experiential learning and being coached	Often short and variable introductory training given in-house
	Mutual contractual agreement made following detailed first interview matching methods and expertise	Mutual contractual agreement made based on practitioner experience and expectations
	Coaches expected to have ongoing supervision as a requirement of their Ethical Code (EMCC 2004)	Supervisors expected to have ongoing supervision as best practice
	Coaching working towards becoming regulated that will include supervision as a professional requirement	No regulation of clinical supervisors although clinical practice regulated as a professional activity
	Coaching as an emerging profession in its own right	Supervision viewed as an additional part of a qualified practitioner's role
	Always an emphasis on client solutions and results for the immediate future	Often an emphasis on 'problems' and 'problem-solving' occurring in practice
Co-creating the relationship	Client/coach agree terms and fees	Free at the point of delivery
	Process mainly based on individual telephone conversations	Process mainly based on 'face-to-face' encounters either individually or as a group
	Coach often external to the organization	Supervisor often internal to the organization

TABLE 6.1 *(cont'd)*

	COACHINIG	CLINICAL SUPERVISION
	Short- to medium-term relationship Coaching viewed as adding value to the organization in developing key staff	Medium- to longer-term relationship Clinical supervision aimed at all healthcare professionals, particularly inexperienced staff
Communicating effectively	Tendency to be non-directive as a coach The client is the expert in the conversation based on their situation Coach suspends experience and expertise unless client gives permission Clarity with coaching role and expectations	Tendency to be more directive as a supervisor Tendency for the supervisor to be an expert in the conversation Supervisor often uses professional experience and expertise in the meeting Sometimes confusion with supervisory role and expectations
Facilitating learning and results	Always an emphasis on client response-ability during and after session Emphasis on the person's performance and life as a client Coaching evaluated through outcomes and results produced by the client	Often an emphasis on supervisee professional accountability during and after session Emphasis on supervisee professional performance at work Difficulty in evaluating the effectiveness of supervision

A major difference is that clinical supervision is seen as an additional part of a practitioner's role following some introductory training but the newly adopted role (if it is adopted) does not relieve the practitioner of existing clinical responsibilities and often no additional time is built in for the activity. In contrast, most coaches have undergone lengthy periods of experiential training to become accredited before practising as a paid professional. While coaching is viewed as adding value to the organization through the individualized development of staff, clinical supervision, which has a similar philosophy, is often viewed as an inconvenience in busy practice.

Both the coaching and clinical supervision literature distance themselves from being any form of therapy, preferring instead to concentrate on the client's or supervisee's 'present' practices. As O'Donovan & Martin (2000:13) assert:

> Unlike therapies, coaching focuses on where you are now and where you want to get to, and the only place you can start from is where you are now.

While professional coaching has an established knowledge base derived from counselling, management consulting and psychology (Hadikin 2004, Peltier 2001, Starr 2003, West & Milan 2001), clinical supervision is only just beginning to explore different psychological frameworks as being relevant for clinical supervisors (discussed in an earlier chapter). This might explain why clinical supervision still largely remains a 'problem'-orientated intervention — not dissimilar to a medical model in which patient problems (practice problems) are identified in order to help diagnose a condition (why such problems are occurring), before a treatment plan is prescribed (action plan to solve the problem — and if not followed through, creates even more problems).

By contrast (in not adopting a negative fault-finding approach), professional coaching is a focused activity that adopts a more appreciative or positive approach concentrating on creating solutions and results with the client. Embracing a similar approach in the clinical supervision encounter could be transformational by creating deeper self-awareness in supervisees about their practice and focusing on improvement and change as an outcome. In turn, this will make the process more transparent and evaluating the effectiveness of clinical supervision less challenging, which is the subject of a later chapter.

While it is not our suggestion that coaching replaces clinical supervision, some key elements of development coaching can quite easily be adapted for use in the clinical supervision situation, particularly with more senior healthcare practitioners (Driscoll & Cooper 2005). However, this will mean re-negotiating the original clinical supervision intentions and expectations with the supervisee. Despite these obvious differences, coaching in my view shares more similarities than differences with clinical supervision:

- The terms coaching and supervision can evoke initial suspicion in the client/supervisee that they are suspected of underperforming.

- Client/supervisee can exercise choice in who is their coach/supervisor.

- Formal contract/agreement is made at the beginning of the process.

- Expectation that the client/supervisee is in control of the process.

- Senior managers can be coaches/supervisors.

- Both processes are examples of formalized reflection geared to developing personal practice and improving performance.

- Sessions begin with present practice and are directed towards future actions.

- Reflective questioning and active listening are key tools used by the coach/supervisor.

- Both processes offer feedback to the client/supervisee.

- Coaches/supervisors are expected to have on going supervision as part of their continuing professional development (CPD).

- Both processes are intended to contribute to the personal and professional growth of the client/supervisee.

Coaching is an eclectic discipline and draws on many sources of knowledge, including research findings and discussions in psychological literature. Using this experience from the world of coaching, some key areas could be further developed in clinical supervision training:

- placing more emphasis on the use of powerful questions,

- active listening,

- designing actions with the supervisee during the session, and

- a willingness to embrace a more holistic approach that takes account of the personal as well as the professional life of the person.

It is interesting to contrast the commitment of the supervisee and the supervisor in clinical supervision, which is 'given freely' in the NHS, to the commitment of the client who pays for individual sessions or is sponsored by their organization to engage in coaching to maximize their performance at work. Finally, all coaching and clinical supervision is concerned with the personal or professional growth of the person and a powerful metaphor comes to mind that explains the complex nature of both coaching and clinical supervision's part in this growth — The Rose (cited by Wright 1998:186).

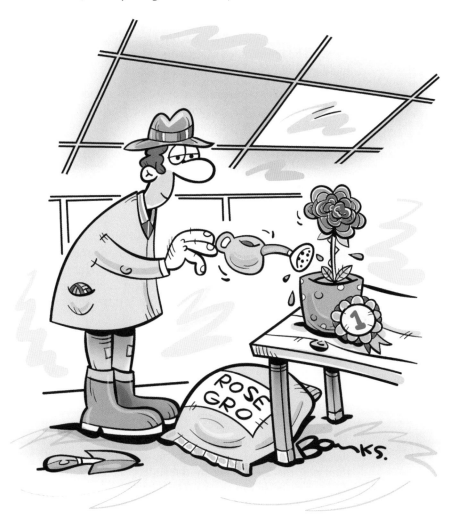

When we plant a rose seed in the earth, we notice that it is small, but we do not criticize it as 'rootless' or 'stemless'. We treat it as a seed, giving it the water and nourishment required of a seed. When it first shoots out of the earth, we don't condemn it as 'immature' or 'underdeveloped', nor do we criticize the buds for not being open when they appear. We stand in wonder at the process taking place and give the plant the care that it needs at each stage of its growth. The rose is a rose from the time it is a seed to the time that it dies. Within it, at all times, it contains its whole potential. It seems to be constantly in the process of change, yet at each state, at each moment, it is perfectly alright as it is.

EXPERIMENTING WITH A COACHING FRAMEWORK IN THE CLINICAL SUPERVISION SITUATION

Clinical supervision, like coaching, relies on the sessions being productive for the supervisee. One way of achieving this is to use a framework or structure to help you navigate your way through a session as a clinical supervisor. Within the coaching literature there are many frameworks to choose from but the most widely used is the GROW model (West & Milan 2001:19). Originally developed by Graham Alexander in 1984 it was published by Sir John Whitmore in his seminal coaching text *Coaching for Performance* (Whitmore 1992). The importance of growth (of the client) is a critical element of coaching highlighted by the following definitions:

> … a simple yet effective form of personal development where the client and coach create an alliance that promotes and sustains the client's personal growth and competence.
> European Coaching Institute, 2006b

> Coaching is about performing at your best through the individual and private assistance of someone who will challenge, stimulate and guide you to keep growing.
> O'Donovan, 2006

The framework John has been using on his coaching course and experimenting with in clinical supervision is the slightly adapted TGROW model (Downey 1999:29) diagrammatically represented in Figure 6.1. As part of the initial clinical supervision agreement a clinical supervisor is expected to control the structure and process of a meeting but it is the supervisee who controls the content or *topic*.

 If you are going to try out the TGROW framework in your next clinical supervision session you will need to seek permission to do so from your supervisor first!

The supervisee's chosen topic for discussion in clinical supervision (while this is seemingly obvious) is critical to the overall outcome of the session. More often than not, the agenda set by the supervisee can have several layers that can be difficult to tease out even under questioning. Therefore, to make the sessions more effective the supervisee should be asked to carry out some written preparation beforehand. (Coaching is frequently carried out on a telephone and this is dealt with in more detail in the next chapter.)

It is often helpful for the supervisee to have begun to reflect on what is to be discussed and to have either emailed or faxed a preparation document to the clinical supervisor beforehand. (The format for this can be discussed when the initial agreement is being negotiated.) Such groundwork is useful in giving the clinical supervisor time to prepare for the session.

Some ideas for questions a clinical supervisor might pose (although not all need to be used; you can probably think of others) using a TGROW framework in a clinical supervision session are contained in Box 6.4.

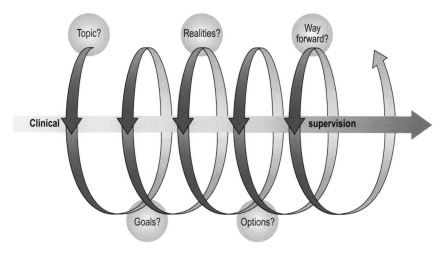

Figure 6.1 A continuous spiral diagram

Obviously it is less intrusive to have questions in front of you when using the telephone than in the face-to-face encounter, but it is surprising how quickly TGROW can be used once you are familiar with its different elements.

As already mentioned, therapy is different from clinical supervision and coaching in that a goal to aim for is established *before* the client/supervisee's actual realities are examined. But, the setting of a positive goal may have little meaning for a client/supervisee who is overwhelmed with the perceived negative

BOX 6.4	*Questions using the TGROW framework a clinical supervisor might pose to a supervisee to aid structure and focus a clinical supervision session*

TOPIC

- What is it you would like to discuss today?
- What issue is uppermost in your mind from your preparation for the session?
- What is the topic or agenda for the session today?

GOAL

- By the time your hand hits the door-handle at the end of the session …what would you like to have achieved?
- What would you like to be different when you leave the session today?
- If I could grant you a wish for today's session, what would it be?

REALITY

- What is happening to you at the moment?
- How do know this to be accurate?
- Can you give me a worked example over the last week when this happens?
- What effect does this have on you?

| BOX 6.4 | *(cont'd)* |

- What seems to be preventing you from making progress?
- What have you tried so far?
- What support or resources might you be able to draw on with your situation?

OPTIONS

- Can you write down six things that you could do right now (however improbable) to improve your situation?
- What resources do you have at your disposal to alter your situation?
- What might be some of the benefits and burdens of each of your ideas?
- Which idea would give you the most happiness in your situation?
- What are the possibilities for your future actions (do not all need to be realistic at this stage)?
- Who might be able to help you with this?
- Would you like some suggestions from me (if client/supervisee stuck)?
- Could you rate from 0 to 5 the practicalities of each of your suggestions?

WAY FORWARD

- What are you now going to do?
- What will your first step(s) be based on today's session?
- When will you begin?
- What might get in your way and how will you deal with this?
- How are you going to remember what you have agreed to do by the time we next meet?
- How will you get the support to move forward?
- Would you be agreeable to email or telephone me about your progress before we next meet?

realities of the present work situation and this can have an influence on the effectiveness of a session. Thus, in clinical supervision, a session is often 'problem driven' instead of being more positive and solution focused, as is the case in coaching. That is why clinical supervision can benefit from adopting the processes involved in coaching: goals that are formed by looking at the situation in the longer term and determining the steps needed to be taken to achieve these goal(s) are motivating and creative for the client/supervisee. In addition to this, setting goals provides not only focus but a way of being able to evaluate the effectiveness of the session based on goal outcomes.

However, keeping in mind the ease with which clinical supervision can fall into a 'problem-driven' session, to be able to successfully achieve client/supervisee goals it is important to do a *reality* check of the client/supervisee situation. This is a critical phase for the coach/supervisor to help the coach/supervisee assess the impact of those realities. Being a neutral or objective listener can help the client/supervisee reframe their situation or view it from a fresh perspective.

An often asked question is: Can someone from outside a professional discipline act as a clinical supervisor? John's own experience is that it is much easier to be objective when you do not fully understand the supervisee's realities or situation and this gives you a license as a supervisor to ask 'silly questions' that get right to the heart of the matter (Sood & Driscoll 2004).

Another important element of helping the client/supervisee with their realities as a coach/supervisor is to remain 'in the present' with the intention of enabling movement forward on the topic. Here using open-ended questions is useful. Sometimes questions can be purposely structured to move the client/supervisee back into 'today' with a view to 'tomorrow' rather than remaining stuck in 'yesterday'! Although the 'past' might be useful to understand the context of a situation, coaching/clinical supervision is not therapy. And sometimes talking about the past can be an unconscious ploy to avoid facing present reality; the supervisor should remain aware of these pitfalls.

The *options* phase helps to develop a sense of personal ownership of the issue and encourage choice, once a path has been cleared through the jungle of the client/supervisee's reality. If the previous phase has been rushed or inadequate time given for detailed questioning, it will reduce those choices and subsequent decision-making by the client/supervisee. Sometimes in exploring options it becomes obvious that more work needs to be done in the initial goal setting or gaining clarity about the client/supervisee's reality. A key element of this stage is to develop a real sense of the client/supervisee's ownership by facilitating as many choices or options as possible to move forward, rather than it being a phase in which the 'right' answer must be found. The more courses of action the client/supervisee generates, the more likely it is that they will be able to change their perspective of the situation and raise some positive energy, enabling progress to be made with their topic.

A critical success factor in clinical supervision and coaching is the development of a safe and confidential environment in which to explore ideas. The generation of options can be limited if the coach/supervisor pours cold water on ideas being produced because they have an in-depth knowledge of the client/supervisee's situation (for example, working in the same environment). Therefore, it could be claimed that in contrast to a clinical supervisor, a neutral observer, such as a coach, offers the client/supervisee the big advantage of an unbiased perspective that allows the exploration of even the most unlikely of ideas.

The *way forward* is the final stage of the process that enables the client/supervisee to convert their images and discussions into decisive actions. This means that the client/supervisee makes final choices and decisions about how to progress. (At this point, a key responsibility, the coach/supervisor summarizes the session, which assists the client/supervisee to come to decisions. This is where it can be of benefit (with permission), for the coach/supervisor to have taken some notes.)

 Taking notes is more awkward in the face-to-face encounter, where in doing so you may stand accused of not actively listening! On a telephone it is much easier, provided you have a headset on which you can listen while you write.

The final phase is where the client/supervisee then needs to demonstrate a commitment to act or be response-able. The session ends with the client/supervisee agreeing the steps that will be taken, how these will be taken, and that they *will* be taken. Most coaches will have been taught (and both myself and Gerard have been on the receiving end of this) to *nail down* the client at the end of each session by asking the client/supervisee to rate three questions on a score of 1 (definitely not) to 10 (definitely will):

- How strong is your *intention* to take that first step?
- How high is your *enthusiasm* for taking that first step?
- How strong is your *commitment* to taking that first step?

Experience suggests that scoring 7 or less on each of these is likely to mean that little or no action will be taken following the session. The language used by the client/supervisee in response to the questions is often just as important as the verbal score. Low intention words such as 'perhaps', 'might' and 'if' can be indicators of intending to act or not after the session.

While the TGROW framework is the most widely known and used in coaching, there are other models that you might wish to explore as an alternative framework for clinical supervision (Dembkowski & Eldridge 2003, Leibling & Prior 2003, Libri 2004, Mackintosh 2003, Martin 2001, Somers 2002). Rushing the stages (because of the lack of time or the inexperience in its use) limits the effectiveness of the TGROW framework. For instance, this may lead to skipping through the stages, and not having a full understanding of the goal(s) representing the gap between the present situation and the desired outcomes or, when generating options, only highlighting a few 'tried and tested' choices. Despite such limitations, in my experience TGROW does provide an excellent structure for those new to coaching but more importantly, it is enormously helpful in clinical supervision.

COACHING POSSIBILITIES IN UK HEALTHCARE BEYOND CLINICAL SUPERVISION

According to The Coaching Study (Arnott & Sparrow 2004) involving over 100 UK organizations (including eight NHS organizations), a significant increase in the use of externally facilitated coaching is predicted in the near future. At present the majority of professional coaching is provided at executive/management levels and concerned with supporting both personal and professional development to improve organizational performance. With the emphasis on ensuring that staff continuing professional development needs are met in clinical governance (McSherry & Pearce 2002, Swage 2003), the potential for coaching still remains relatively unexplored as a tool for developing health professionals' practice.

Although coaching might be viewed as a tool for empowering individuals (Hughes 2003), great coaches know that individuals already have innate power and potential so therefore a coach's task is to facilitate expression of it (Downey 1999:13). While this chapter has concentrated on the use of coaching as a method for clinical supervision, Hadikin (2004) outlines a powerful case for developing a whole coaching culture in the NHS with a broader application to healthcare and in particular to patients:

... as we move as a society from a sickness/cure model towards a health/
prevention model, we should look towards a profession which facilitates
growth and change rather than a therapeutic model to 'cure' our 'illness'.
Hadikin, 2004:24

Hughes (2003) suggests that coaching, where the client (or the supervisee) is
promoted or empowered to see themselves as being an expert in their own
situation, can be applied with patients. Current government initiatives are doing
just that, promoting the patient as an expert in their own experience of illness
(Department of Health 2001). Imagine the vast resources that might be saved if
healthcare staff were able to coach patients with chronic conditions to take
more control over their lives rather than be dependent on a healthcare system
that would seem to favour acute illness. Some evidence is already emerging that
coaching can have a favourable effect on patient outcomes (Boyle 2004, Brook
et al 2003, Horowitz et al 2002, Hughes 2003, Ream et al 2002, Vale et al
2003, Whittemore et al 2001, Whyte 1997). While a coaching potential for
developing healthcare staff in clinical supervision is a distinct possibility, an
even greater potential for developing a coaching culture generally in UK healthcare could emerge. Perhaps development coaching might even become the new
clinical supervision.

CONCLUSION

The historical development of sporting coaching techniques and psychological processes has moved rapidly from the playing field to transforming the performances
of individuals and organizations in corporate business. The professional coaching
knowledge that coaches use is only now beginning to be realized in healthcare
and, like clinical supervision was, and perhaps still is, is poorly understood.

While I am not advocating development coaching as a replacement for clinical
supervision or all clinical supervision to become development coaching, there
would seem to be an enormous potential for the principles of professional coaching in clinical supervision as well as in the healthcare setting generally. The processes of both clinical supervision and development coaching seem to support
the personal and professional growth of the 'client' or 'supervisee'. The way that
this is achieved is through regular reflective but action-orientated conversations
intended to increase future performance as a person and a practitioner. Unlike
clinical supervision, which undoubtedly has supervisee outcomes, development
coaching is more transparent while remaining confidential. It is less 'problem'
orientated than clinical supervision and has at its core demonstrable results following a structured conversation that increase professional performance, making
a positive contribution to the client's personal wellbeing. The key is that all parties develop an understanding about the intentions and expectations beforehand
or when periodically re-negotiating the coaching or clinical supervision agreement or contract.

For those reading this chapter as professional coaches we extend an invitation and point out the potential 'alliance' that could exist between healthcare
and coaching. Perhaps some of the lessons and expertise of developing clinical
supervision in UK healthcare over the last decade might offer the emerging

profession of coaching a way forward that requires practising coaches to also engage in 'regular' supervision as part of their continuing professional development (CPD) (or might this be development coaching?).

On reflection . . . chapter summary

- Professional coaching remains an unexplored frontier for the continued development of clinical supervision in healthcare
- The term 'development coaching' might be a more accurate description of clinical supervision for more senior healthcare practitioners
- Unlike for professional coaching there is an absence of literature and virtually no agreement on what the core competencies of a clinical supervisor are
- Both clinical supervision and professional coaching have as their cores the facilitation of a reflective conversation with another person to enhance their personal and professional growth
- Professional coaching frameworks are less 'problem' orientated and can offer structure for achieving demonstrable outcomes in clinical supervision

FURTHER READING

Gallwey W T 1986 The inner game of tennis. Pan Books, London

Hargrove R 2003 Masterful coaching (revised edn). Jossey Bass/Pfeiffer, San Francisco, CA, USA

Hargrove R 2003 Masterful coaching fieldbook. Jossey Bass/Pfeiffer, San Francisco, CA, USA

Harrold F 2000 Be your own life coach. Hodder & Stoughton, London

Flaherty J 1999 Coaching evoking excellence in others. Butterworth-Heinemann (Elsevier), Burlington MA, USA

Kline N 1999 Time to think – listening to ignite the human mind ward lock. London

Landsberg M 1996 The TAO of coaching. Harper-Collins, London

Leonard T 1998 The portable coach. Scribner, New York

Neenan M, Dryden W 2002 Life coaching: a cognitive behavioural approach. Brunner-Routledge, East Sussex, UK

Robbins A 2001 Awaken the giant within. Pocket Books. Simon & Schuster, London, UK

Robbins A 2001 Notes from a friend. Pocket Books. Simon & Schuster, London, UK

Von Oech R 1990 A whack on the side of the head: how you can be more creative. Thorsons, London

Whitworth L, Kimsey-House H, Sandahl P 1988 Co-active coaching: new skills for coaching people toward success in work and life. Davies-Black, CA, USA

Yeung R 2000 Coaching people. How To Books, Oxford

Zeus P, Skiffington S 2001 The complete guide to coaching at work. MacGraw Hill, Australia

SELECTED COACHING WEBSITE/RESOURCES

http://www.academyofexecutivecoaching.co.uk
http://www.associationforcoaching.com
http://www.coachfederation.org/
http://www.coachinc.com
http://www.supervisionandcoaching.com
http://www.coachingnetwork.org.uk
http://www.24-7coaching.com
http://coachueurope.com
http://www.coachville.com
http://www.lifecoaching-company.co.uk
http://www.noble-manhattan.com
http://www.oscm.com
http://www.performance-am.com/coaching_articles.htm
http://www.pmcscotland.com
http://www.solutionbox.com
http://www.theinnergame.com

REFERENCES

Anderson R H, Snyder K J (eds) 1993 Clinical supervision – coaching for higher performance. Technomic, Pennysylvania, USA

Arnott J, Sparrow J 2004 The coaching study 2004. University of Central England (UCE), Birmingham, UK

Association for Coaching 2005 Supervision report. Online. Available at: http://www.associationforcoaching.com/about/ACSuper.doc Accessed 1/7/06

Boyle D 2004 Coaching for recovery: a key mental health skill. Life in the Day 8(1):23–27

Brook O, Van Hout H, Nieuwenhuysea H et al 2003 Effects of coaching by community pharmacists on psychological symptoms of antidepressant users; a randomised controlled trial. European Neuropsychopharmacology 13:347–354

Dembkowski S, Eldridge F 2003 Beyond GROW: a new coaching model. The International Journal of Mentoring and Coaching 1(1):(November)

Department of Health 2001 The expert patient: a new approach to chronic disease management. Stationery Office, London

Downey M 1999 Effective coaching. Orion Business Books, London

Driscoll J J, Cooper R 2005 Coaching for clinicians. Nursing Management 12(1): 18–23

ECI 2006a Europe's Accreditation Body for Coaches and Coach Training Providers. Online. Available at: http://www.europeancoachinginstitute.org/about_eci/. Accessed 23/4/06

ECI 2006b What is coaching? What is coaching about? Online. Available at: http://www.europeancoachinginstitute.org/what_is_coaching/. Accessed 23/4/06

EMCC 2004a European Mentoring and Coaching Council code of ethics. Online. Available at: http://www.emccouncil.org/

Downloads/EMCC_Code_of_Ethics.pdf. Accessed 4/10/04

EMCC 2004b European Mentoring and Coaching Council guidelines for supervision. Available at: http://www.emccouncil.org/ Downloads/EMCC_Guidelines_On_ Supervision.PDF. Accessed 10/9/04

Gallwey W T 2000 The inner game of work. 2nd edn. Orion Business Books, London

Hadikin R 2004 Effective coaching in healthcare. Books for Midwives, Elsevier, Oxford, UK

Horowitz J, Bell M, Trybulski J 2002 Promoting responsiveness between mothers with depressive symptoms and their infants. Journal of Nursing Scholarship 33(4):323–329

Hughes S 2003 Promoting independence: the nurse as coach. Nursing Standard 18(10):42–44

ICF (International Coach Federation) 2006a The ICF (UK) code of ethics. The ICF Definition of Coaching. Online. Available at: http://www.coachfederation.org.uk/ introducing_icf/icf_code_of_ethics.phtml. Accessed 23/4/06

ICF (International Coach Federation) 2006b The ICF (UK) coaching core competencies. Online. Available at: http://www.coachfederation.org.uk/gaining _the_icfs_professional_qualification/coachi ng_core_competencies.phtml. Accessed 23/4/06

Jarvis J 2004 Coaching and buying coaching services. Chartered Institute of Personnel and Development (CIPD), London

Jay M 2001 Distinguishing coaching practice arenas. Organisations & People 8(4):19–25

Kinlaw D C 1997 Coaching – winning strategies for individuals and teams. Gower, Hampshire, UK

Leibling M, Prior R 2003 Coaching made easy. Kogan Page, London

Libri V 2004 Beyond GROW: in search of acronyms and coaching models. The International Journal of Mentoring and Coaching 2(1).

Mackintosh A 2003 Using the Outcomes Coaching System and Carers™ to enhance management and employee performance. Performance Management Coaching (PMC), Glasgow, Scotland

McSherry R, Pearce P 2002 Clinical governance a guide to implementation for healthcare professionals. Blackwell, London

Martin C 2001 The life coaching handbook. Crown House, Carmarthen, Wales

O'Donovan G, Martin C 2000 The thirty minute life coach. The Coaching Academy, Portsmouth, UK

O'Donovan, G 2006 A definition of life coaching.Online. Available at: http://www.noble-manhattan.com/ coach_training/what_is_life_coaching/defin ition_of_coaching/. Accessed 23/4/06

Peltier B 2001 The psychology of executive coaching. Brunner-Routledge (Taylor & Francis Group), East Sussex, UK

Ream E, Richardson A, Alexander-Dann C 2002 Facilitating patients' coping with fatigue during chemotherapy – pilot outcomes. Cancer Nursing 25(4):300–308

Somers M 2002 Coaching in a week. Hodder & Stoughton, London

Sood A, Driscoll J 2004 Clinical supervision in practice: a working model. Macmillan Voice (29) Spring (pull out-supplement), Macmillan Cancer Relief

Starr J 2003 The coaching manual. Prentice Hall Business, London

Swage T 2003 Clinical governance in healthcare practice. 2nd edn. Butterworth-Heinemann, London

Thorpe S, Clifford J 2003 The coaching handbook: an action kit for trainers and managers. Kogan Page, London

UKCLC 2003 The future of coaching – prospects and challenges for life. Coaching Life College Press / UK College of Life Coaching, Wolverhampton, UK

Vale M, Jelinek M, Best J et al (COACH Study Group) 2003 Coaching patients on achieving cardiovascular health (COACH): a multicenter randomized trial in patients with coronary heart disease. Archives of Internal Medicine 22(163):2775–2783

West L, Milan M 2001 The reflecting glass – professional coaching for leadership development. Palgrave, Basingstoke, UK

Whitmore J 1992 Coaching for performance. Nicholas-Brearley, London

Whittemore J, Chase S, Mandle C 2001 The integrity and efficacy of a nurse-coaching intervention in type 2 diabetes. The Diabetes Educator 27:887–898

Whyte L 1997 Coaching for change: realising the potential for nursing. Nursing Management 3(10):12–13

Wright K 1998 Breaking the rules – removing the obstacles to effortless high performance. CPM, ID, USA

7 Alternative methods in clinical supervision: beyond the face-to-face encounter

John Driscoll and Allan Townsend

INTRODUCTION

As has already been outlined in previous chapters, while organizational support does exist for the development of clinical supervision, particularly in UK healthcare, there remain significant challenges in its widespread implementation. Factors such as health professional resistance and being viewed as a low-priority activity, time constraints, staff shortages, access to appropriate supervisors and finding a suitable environment in which to discuss practice issues present significant challenges in even getting started at all.

Such factors are magnified when the implementation of clinical supervision (or indeed any new initiative) requires practitioners talking on a regular basis across vast distances, such as those found in the remote rural areas of Australia. Here, as in other countries of great land distances, there has been a need for lateral thinking to be undertaken to find solutions to such challenges and to develop alternative methods and formats for the delivery of clinical supervision (Crago & Crago 2002, Milne & Oliver 2000) that cannot be effectively carried out in a face-to-face situation.

Significant improvements in technology and a growing awareness and familiarity with its usage for clinical supervision are already beginning to meet that challenge of distance. It could be argued that the advent of technological innovations has diminished the practical barriers of 'doing' clinical supervision across great distances, reducing what previously might have been an 'actual' problem to only a 'perceptual' problem. Distance can now be regarded as simply a lame excuse for not getting started. Once again, as has often been pointed out in this book, there is no need for healthcare professionals to re-invent the wheel; they but need to look to other disciplines (or countries) that are taking things forward by utilizing technology as an adjunct to the development of clinical supervision.

The title of our chapter probably reflects the mainstream view that for many healthcare professionals the use of technology, although it represents an 'alternative way' of getting going with clinical supervision, has yet to establish itself as a practical complementary method. Allan, using his experience of working on the railways in Australia prior to becoming a mental health nurse, provides a powerful metaphor:

> ... Coming from a railway industry background, I liken the 'getting going with clinical supervision' issue to freight trains. A freight train is made up of an engine (for instance a supervisee) and has numerous loaded wagons (baggage/issues for clinical supervision) that is faced with the task of hauling its load to a destination point to be unloaded (resolving or airing an issue with the clinical supervisor). If the track is on a slight decline and free of barriers then 'getting going' on the journey is relatively easy, only requiring a minimum amount of effort. On the other hand, if the track is on an incline with a number of barriers to overcome (distance, fatigue and finding the time for clinical supervision) then extra effort or support may be required to get, or even keep going. In this instance in railway terms, a bank engine or 'banker' is used to provide that extra effort required to assist the freight train until it is clear of its uphill climb. Experimenting with alternative methods of clinical supervision could act as the 'banker' just as like with the freight train that helps remove, or significantly reduce the impact of 'real' or 'perceived' barriers to 'getting going' (in clinical supervision) ...

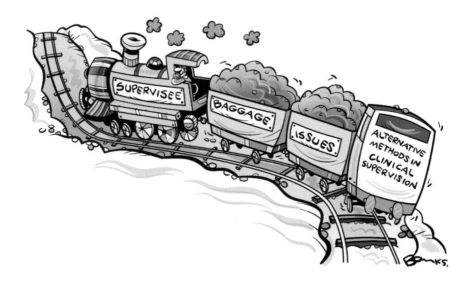

For those of you who are facing some of those barriers to getting started with clinical supervision already outlined, our challenge is: reflect on some of the benefits, as well as some of the burdens, of using technology and decide whether using that technology to provide clinical supervision is better than not having any clinical supervision at all.

Kate Anthony opens the doors of possibility for alternative methods of clinical supervision in healthcare in her pioneering work on counselling and psychotherapy when she states:

> What is clear, once we get over our fears of using technology (in counselling and psychotherapy), is that we are examining the same phenomenon that has happened in all types of therapy in the last 100 years: the fact that communication between two parties is the key to finding mental well being in the face of our life circumstance. We are still human beings interacting with each other to try to cope with problems; we are just communicating using a different set of tools.
> Anthony, 2003:15

Anthony (2003:15) also provides a helpful classification of the technologies currently available for use in clinical supervision:

- a purely auditory experience of each other (use of the telephone),
- with visual and audio experience taking place at a distance (video conferencing),
- without any visual or audio experience of each other (as when communication is exclusively by text — such as internet chat or electronic mail),
- with remote visual and audio experience taking place (computer-assisted therapy programmes).

The purpose of this chapter is to help you explore the use of the telephone, video conferencing and computerized text to allow you make up your own mind about whether these technologies might suit your own clinical supervision situation or not. Although we will not be exploring computer-assisted therapy programmes for use in clinical supervision, more detailed accounts of these programmes can be found in Cavanagh et al (2003a, 2003b). The sections in this chapter, which you can dip in and out of, are intended not only to offer our first-hand experiences with the use of the telephone and video conferencing in clinical supervision, but also to share the work of others who have used, and continue to research, computerized methods in clinical supervision, particularly in mental health arenas.

We hope that reading this will give you practical ideas and the courage to experiment with technology as an alternative experience for clinical supervision where the face-to-face encounter is not available, or simply to validate its potential for you in practice. We conclude that whilst the face-to-face encounter in clinical supervision might currently be the preferred method for clinical supervision in healthcare, in our joint experiences, it is unlikely that it will remain the only viable method for much longer.

SOME INITIAL THOUGHTS ABOUT THE POTENTIAL IMPACT OF TECHNOLOGY IN CLINICAL SUPERVISION

The scope of technology that an individual (or an organization) can utilize is vast, for example, a personal computer with a word processor, a mobile phone with multimedia functions or the latest state-of-the-art computerized communication systems where it is possible to link individuals or groups across the globe.

Regardless of the complexity of the system or the size of the organization, the incorporation of information technology systems will be accompanied by the need to change or alter older, perhaps preferred, ways of working. The same argument could apply to the future of clinical supervision. Perhaps the preferred face-to-face encounter is becoming challenged by the increasing opportunities to independently network across distance, reducing the need to even move out of the office or home to obtain clinical supervision. The application of information and communications technology in clinical supervision offers distinct advantages as well as challenges. However, it is worth remembering that the different technologies are simply methods to get going with clinical supervision and not the process itself. In other words, whatever technology is used, the process for clinical supervision will remain largely unchanged.

We wonder how many of you reading this have contemplated the thought of using technology to assist you, either getting started with clinical supervision or as an alternative method to what you are currently doing? Perhaps for some of you, the challenges of utilizing technology actually act as a further barrier to getting started in clinical supervision.

Looking at Table 7.1, how do some of our ideas behind the challenges of using advances in information and communications technology in clinical supervision compare to yours?

Thinking about your own situation in clinical supervision, would some of the opportunities outweigh the likely challenges presented by the use of information and communications technology?

What do you think might be the implications of this in your own practice arena?

While the range of information and communication technologies is vast, increasing in complexity and often expensive to use, one technology that is often taken for granted (or perhaps not even included as a technology) for clinical supervision is the telephone.

USING THE TELEPHONE FOR INDIVIDUAL AND GROUP CLINICAL SUPERVISION

The telephone remains one of the cheapest and simplest technologies and is used extensively in many forms of counselling and psychotherapy (Copeland 2003, Rosenfield 2003, Sanders 1996) and professional coaching (Hadikin 2004, Mackintosh 2005), so why not in clinical supervision?

As with the face-to-face encounter, before commencing a new method of clinical supervision it is important to agree a contract to establish what is expected of all parties. Based on Rosenfield's (1997:101) original work and our personal experiences of using the one-to-one telephone method for clinical supervision across continents, reasons are outlined in Box 7.1 as to why a telephone method might be preferable for clinical supervision.

Might some of the reasons listed influence your thinking on the adoption of the telephone method for your own clinical supervision?

TABLE 7.1 *Some challenges and opportunities utilizing information and communications technology in clinical supervision*

Challenges	Opportunities
Reduced body language signals to read and interpret, e.g. lack of visual clues	Less fatigue and expense incurred by travelling to supervision meetings
More difficult to gain rapport and develop trust where there are no visual clues	Increased accessibility to a wider range of potential clinical supervisors
Development of listening skills and other strategies for reading 'e' language	Geographical distance for clinical supervision meetings less of a problem
Increased preparation prior to method being employed	Easier retrieval of session notes to remember issues discussed and action points agreed
Issues around confidentiality and possibility of retrieval of recorded materials at a later date	More ability and freedom to express emotions with someone you cannot see
Less spontaneity than in face-to-face conversations, e.g. having to wait turns, knowing when to intervene	Clinical supervision can seem more 'equal' and increased levels of control for the supervisee in what is happening
Development of new 'e' supervisory skills	New skills learned with using technology in clinical supervision, e.g. active listening can be applied in a range of other situations
Uncomfortable in embarking on new forms of clinical supervision	More acceptable for participants to take notes whilst the session is ongoing
Unsure about some of the key differences in contracting for clinical supervision using technological methods	Quicker trusting relationships developed with a clinical supervisor you have not seen
Personal difficulties in articulating with words	Shorter time required for clinical supervision sessions as meetings more focused and productive than in face-to-face encounters
Feelings of potential awkwardness in dealing with silences or gaps in conversations	Clinical supervision using new methods and formats can be an experiential learning experience for all concerned
Self-consciousness about appearance replaced by concerns about use of technology	Reduced worries about body language being interpreted and general appearance
Clinical supervision can occur outside the immediate workplace and intrude on home and social life	Increased need to pay attention to contracting in clinical supervision in methods you may be unfamiliar with
Prior plans made for clinical supervision meetings to occur over distance are reliant on whatever system is employed for it to work effectively	It is not always necessary to be in a traditional work environment for clinical supervision to happen

 While there seem to be potential advantages to using the one-to-one telephone method, can you think of times when the telephone might not be appropriate or suitable in clinical supervision?

BOX 7.1	*Some reasons why a one-to-one telephone method might be preferable to the face-to-face method*

- Wider geographical range and remote access to supervisors/supervisees
- Preference to work in a particular orientation that might not be available locally
- Removes the need to physically travel to meetings
- Ecologically friendly
- Cost-efficient due to reduced transport costs
- Neither has to be 100% fit to participate in a meeting
- Greater equality in a telephone relationship, where one party can terminate at any time simply by hanging up
- More easy to challenge someone you cannot see
- More need to check assumptions as four of the five senses are not used when talking on the telephone (the voice being the only clue)
- Might increase clinical supervision uptake within organizations by being a more flexible method
- The tendency not to take for granted planned telephone calls by preparing more thoroughly than when in the face-to-face situation
- Increased possibilities for recording conversations to listen to at a later date, although there are implications for the maintenance of confidentiality
- Increased likelihood of being listened to
- Feelings of more privacy and being more safe to talk at work
- Challenges the notion that clinical supervision takes place on *either* the supervisors' *or* the supervisee' terms; it becomes an alliance between both parties

Based on our experience of engaging in international telephone clinical supervision, which happened every month for a year, there are practical realities that need to influence the formation of an initial contract, while other issues which may emerge over time need to be worked through (Box 7.2). Our preliminary contact was through the 'text-based method' of electronic mail (described later in the chapter); this has been reported on by others in clinical supervision literature. However, it soon became obvious that lengthy emails across time zones were not meeting Allan's needs and what was required was a synchronous and active conversation about his practice, based on his struggles to implement clinical supervision in the State of Victoria (which is larger than the the whole of the United Kingdom landmass). This led us to explore different methods of communicating.

The use of the individual telephone method has also been piloted in the UK as a method of clinical supervision to increase accessibility to clinical supervisors for nurses in community settings (Thompson & Winter 2003). Clinical supervisors located in an urban NHS Direct call centre were trained not only in clinical supervision but also in how to use a computer-assisted algorithm with key headings to help the supervisees reflect on their practice. Anonymous compu-

BOX 7.2	*Practical realities to consider for international one-to-one telephone clinical supervision*

- International calls are costly in peak times and require legitimizing with a manager before making international calls in excess of an hour during work time

- Both the supervisee and supervisor need to know international dialling codes and have access to a set landline telephone number for each meeting

- The contractual agreement can help decide how the process will be evaluated *before* clinical supervision commences and be explored using electronic mail before the planned telephone meetings begin

- The contractual agreement will confirm who calls who and when/what happens if a call is missed or should it not be possible to connect the line

- The use of supplementary email support and follow-up in between telephone calls can enhance the impact of telephone clinical supervision

- Talking and actively listening on the telephone in excess of one hour is tiring and challenges the attention span and powers of concentration (our own experience was that as we got used to the method we could do more in less time and reduce the telephone time)

- The telephone needs to be located in a suitable area, e.g. in a private room that is free of distractions and interruptions (e.g. John was always talking on the telephone when the mail arrived in the morning causing the dog to bark and Allan was almost locked in an office working late one evening!)

- Being in familiar surroundings and not directly face-to-face can encourage more challenge to happen

- International time differences (9–10 hours) can mean that while one is at the beginning of their day the other is at the end ... dressing gown or suit?

- It is acceptable to make ongoing notes in a telephone encounter, unlike in face-to-face clinical supervision, although excessive note taking will affect actively listening

- It is useful to use a headset rather than keep holding the telephone for a long time although sound quality can sometimes be affected

- It is an advantage to have met face-to-face prior to beginning telephone clinical supervision

- Auditory clues such as voice, tone, talking style, words, and use of silences are the key tools for active listening and understanding (which was learned as we went along rather than seriously considered before we started — a productive supervisory relationship may depend on listening for verbal clues and cues, particularly if the parties have not met before)

terized data sets or themes from all supervisee telephone meetings (with permission) were collated and fed back to the organization to help with the continual improvement of the service delivery.

While initially the emphasis in telephone clinical supervision has been on the one-to-one encounter, the proportion of work that is undertaken with geographically separated groups of people is significantly increasing (Hogan 2003:377).

Coming from Australia, Allan was already used to the video conferencing method for meetings, but I stated that I thought this might be too expensive for our purposes. Cost being an issue, I remember being dismissive when Allan suggested that he could supply a link up and computer software for us to work with; I was in favour of using a much more familiar and cheaper technology — the telephone!

On reflection, I now acknowledge that my dismissal of the suggestion was probably due to my own anxieties about using a new technology and concerns about falling short of Allan's expectations of me as a competent clinical supervisor. This had acted as a barrier to the use of that method of technology for our own clinical supervision and even today remains an opportunity missed. (Allan pursues the idea later in the chapter.)

Thankfully Allan was undeterred and, after we physically met and worked together in Australia, he set up a team who developed the use of the video conferencing technique as a method of group clinical supervision to support clinical supervisors in rural and remote areas (described in more detail later in the chapter).

Rosenfield (2003:100) suggests that group telephone work provides an excellent medium for short-term work, in which trusting relationships are developed more quickly and fewer sessions are necessary. For clinical supervision in healthcare, the group telephone method has not been widely reported upon, unlike more therapeutic encounters in counselling and psychotherapy; but even in these disciplines, the telephone supervision method often has second class status (Plowman 2003) or is viewed as a stop-gap solution (Copeland 2003) when compared to face-to-face meetings.

When I talk of accessing clinical supervision as a problem for the isolated healthcare professional in the UK, I know that Allan continues to grin to himself as he compares their isolation to the isolation of healthcare professionals in the remote rural areas of some parts of a country the sheer size of Australia.

However, even within the confines of the UK, a need arose to actively support a group of specialist practice development nurses working in Northern Ireland, Wales and England. The Developing Practice Network for practice development nurses, a UK network supported by the charity Foundation of Nursing Studies (www.fons.org), sponsored a project to explore the use of the group telephone method. The full report of that project (Driscoll et al 2006) describes the use of a modified method of action learning (McGill & Beaty 2002) for group telephone clinical supervision (or what is more accurately referred to in the literature as audio teleconferencing). Although facilitating group supervision is dealt with in a later chapter, guidelines for using this form of technology emerged from the project. Some practical hints and tips (Box 7.3) based on our experiential form of learning are offered to those who might wish to consider this method for their own group clinical supervision.

While there are similarities with the practicalities of using the one-to-one telephone clinical supervision method previously described, an additional telephone company facility is required for teleconference to link up all the participants who dial in at a designated time, using a dedicated telephone number and pass numbers. The individual cost of a 90-minute dial in conference for telephone clinical supervision as a group at the time of writing was around 10p a minute, equating to £9 GBP per person per toll-free call (0800) or £90 GBP for

BOX 7.3	*Tips and hints when using telephone clinical supervision (audio teleconferencing) in groups*

Getting organized for the audio conferencing method of clinical supervision:

- Ensure one named person is responsible for liaising with the telephone company to pay the bills, and issue telephone/security numbers for participants to call
- Consider the use of headsets and shoulder rests for lengthy telephone calls
- Consider having a contractual face-to-face meeting beforehand so participants physically see each other first and can discuss ground-rules, e.g. how the meeting will be structured and documented, confidentiality, giving feedback
- Agree the different roles that can be assigned in the meetings such as presenter/supervisee, facilitator(s), peer supervisors, process reviewer or scribe, timekeeper — it is useful to discuss the responsibilities with each role and rotate to experience each of these in the meetings
- Consider what to do with those not in regular attendance or those wishing to join some time later as part of the contracting process
- Think about when is the best time to have the meetings, as active listening and concentrating can be tiring

Before the meeting:

- Always dial in from a landline rather than a mobile or walkabout cordless telephone that will impair sound quality and distract others
- Consider where you intend phoning from, e.g. comfortable, quiet, free from distractions and background noise
- It can be useful for the facilitator/clinical supervisor to dial in a couple of minutes earlier to be able to welcome participants on arrival
- Be on time when dialing in or leave a message if you cannot attend
- If you are to present an issue for clinical supervision, prepare beforehand and try to give a succinct account
- Avoid waiting for participants who may be late and concentrate on those present — get going with the call!
- Ensure everyone can hear each other at the beginning of the call
- Agree the structure, including timing and who will be doing what

During the meeting:

- Speak slower and a bit louder than you would in a face-to-face conversation
- Jot down the names of those participating and make sure everybody has had an opportunity to speak or air an opinion in the meeting
- In the early stages introduce yourself before speaking to the participants
- Briefly review or follow up on the key points of the last meeting before commencing
- A meeting does not have to be brimming with chatter to be effective; participants also need some space or silence to think about their responses

BOX 7.3	*(cont'd)*

- Close the meeting by using a 'round robin' or getting each participant to state something they learned from the meeting or how they are feeling, particularly after sensitive issues have been discussed — when the telephones click off an emptiness will remain

After the meeting:

- Complete any evaluative/reflective documentation as close to the time of the meeting as possible and where appropriate dial in to retrieve archived calls
- If requested by the supervisee, forward further questions by electronic mail for them to be able to reflect on prior to the next meeting
- Ensure you note the time, date and dial-in number of the next meeting
- Consider the personal preparation that will be necessary for the next meeting, e.g. role and responsibilities, confirming attendance or sending apologies, general commitment to the remote group

ten supervisees. The costs were borne out by project monies and did represent value for money, as to meet as a group would have involved flying time for some participants and long rail or car journeys for others. In fact, the whole venture totalled six monthly sessions, all of which were held between 1930 and 2100 hours in the participants' own homes. Additional facilities used by the group were:

- the archiving of each and every call (which could be dialed in using individual security settings if somebody was unable to meet),
- an option of the call being recorded onto a DVD/CD for research purposes (which was not utilized).

Any preliminary web search will reveal that such facilities are often used as a distance learning method, particularly in professional coaching and in the business sector, with numbers as high as 150 participants from around the globe attending an audio conference; however, the rules are different (Hadikin 2004) from the more intimate atmosphere of small group, or individual, telephone supervision.

We would not recommend using group supervision on the telephone with numbers as large as 150; more like 8–10 persons and even less if this is a new method for you!

VIDEO CONFERENCING ACROSS DISTANCE AS COLLABORATIVE CLINICAL SUPERVISION

Video conferencing is a two-way video, audio and sometimes data communication process across long distances between two or more people at different locations in which participants see and hear one another during the interaction

(Motamedi 2001:386). Video conferencing differs from the telephone method by providing the user with live video images in addition to synchronous voice tele-communication, creating the 'virtual reality' of being in the same room with people who may be thousands of miles away. Of all the technological methods available in the business world, video conferencing is considered to bear the closest resemblance to face-to-face communication, as you can do virtually anything in a video conference that you would do in a face-to-face meeting. Diamond (1996) and Simpson (2005) suggest that in a psychotherapy situation therapeutic rela-tionships can be similar to the face-to-face encounter in video conferencing. More detailed reviews of the challenges posed in setting up the video conferencing method in mental health arenas can be found in Capner (2000), Simpson (2003) and Topps (2005).

As with all technology, spending time getting used to the equipment is of paramount importance. Allan always quotes his 6 'Ps' (Prior Preparation and Planning then Prevents Poor Performance) when he talks about video confer-encing and it would seem that this applies not only to the technology but also to the facilitation of it!

… video conferencing is the technology with which you're most likely to have a bad experience. Many groups get over excited with the prospect of what this technology can do for them and the potential cost benefits of eliminating face-to-face meetings. Consequently, too often people rush into video conferencing, neglecting to do the necessary planning, preparation, and facilitation work. The result is often a rather drab and confusing interchange, which turns people off to the technology …
Justice and Jamieson, 1999:416

Don't let technology become a barrier to you getting involved in or continuing in clinical supervision. The key to success when considering the use of video conferencing for clinical supervision is the identification of any gaps in your knowledge and skills, particularly if you are facilitating the event and network with someone who is familiar with the technology already, or accessing the vast amount of information available from the telecom companies themselves. Such companies who manufacture, supply and install video conferencing equipment tend to supply comprehensive manuals which explain how to operate the equipment and troubleshoot it, along with practical tips and discussion on a number of other considerations.

Where might you need to go to get more information about using video conferencing equipment in your work area?

Thinking about the technology available to you where you work, might video conferencing be an option that you would consider using to access clinical supervision?

The use of video conferencing as a medium specifically for clinical supervision is far from new although the advancements in the quality, availability, reliability and cost of the technology have made it vastly different from what it used to be. What is interesting is that (despite some of the seemingly unbearable challenges faced by the early pioneers of video conferencing clinical supervision) people report it to be a success.

Sturmey (1994), in an early research study looking at the use of video conferencing in distance clinical supervision, found that emotional messages, education processes, supervision and relationships could be very successfully carried out provided that any encountered technical problems were not ongoing. The technology at that time provided relatively poor audio and video quality, with delays and poor sequencing between what could be heard and what could be seen. (Some of you might recall early television news bulletins when foreign correspondents reporting from abroad to newsreaders suffered long time delays in feedback, making their conversations stunted and clumsy, and their physical movements often were not aligned with audio, so it was not uncommon for the individuals at both ends of the communication to be unsure of what was happening or being said.) Despite such technological challenges successful interactions in supervision were reported to have taken place. Sturmey (1994) concluded:

> … When technology allows supervision to be carried out from a distance, the positive gain is that specialist skills and knowledge not available in the local area suddenly become available …

Video conferencing now has been immensely refined due to the developments in satellite and cable technology but still it often is seen as a barrier in clinical supervision.

Marrow et al (2002) in a small clinical supervision study for nurses in the UK found that:

> … video conferencing technology was of immense value and helped to reduce the stress and times involved in traveling and promote an active communication between practitioners working in similar specialties but in distance workplace settings …

Interestingly, in the same study a time delay with the technology provided an unexpected supervisory outcome:

> … video conferencing detracted from communication, images/movement were exaggerated and sound was poor … time delay in conversations was inhibitive and didn't enhance supervision … I now feel this encouraged us to listen more intently than normal and wait for the other party to stop before starting a response; perhaps we are all guilty at times of interrupting.
> Marrow et al, 2002:279

Feeling a bit awkward or uncomfortable and learning to adjust is a common experience regardless of the situation, whether it is commencing face-to-face clinical supervision or video conferencing clinical supervision. The reality is that, in time, the clinical supervision session becomes the focal point for the conversation and with experience everything else becomes secondary; meetings or sessions become more structured than normal, focused on the task and less likely to be interrupted than in the face-to-face situation.

My (Allan) experience of international telephone clinical supervision (as previously mentioned by John) was to me surprisingly positive despite the fact that it took me some time to get past the idea that I could not see him, I once thought of getting a photo and putting it on the desk! Despite my conversion to the telephone as a medium for clinical supervision and undeterred by John's lack of confidence in some of the newer technology, together with an enthusiastic group of rural and metropolitan colleagues, I managed to experience video conferencing as a medium for offering clinical supervision to active clinical supervisors. In fairness to John, video conferencing technology is well advanced in Australia, compared to some other countries, and I have the experience, knowledge and, importantly, the confidence to use it. I have also learned quite a bit with this group especially in relation to using video conferencing as a method of clinical supervision.

Following a State Conference in 2003 on Clinical Supervision in Victoria, a clinical supervision programme was developed by Allan and his team and implemented at Ballarat Health Services Psychiatric Services (BHSPS). Prior to 2004, there were very few clinicians at BHSPS that had experienced any formal clinical supervision and therefore the need for ongoing support of clinical supervisors was considered a priority. After some introductory training, follow-up meetings were conducted on a regular basis to allow clinical supervisors to come together and discuss/share their experiences. Clinical supervisors reported that this was supportive and that they could learn from sharing experiences but they also identified the need to tap into the expertise of clinical supervisors from external services due to the lack of exposure and the limited experience of BHSPS clinicians. BHSPS felt that similar gains could be made by exposing some of our clinical supervisors to experienced clinical supervisors from other services, the idea being that those clinical supervisors could enhance their knowledge and skill development and share those experiences with others from within our service.

Getting a video conferencing group together was fortunately a relatively simple process as the technology was not unusual in supporting remote practitioners. Following discussion with metropolitan and rural services, authority was sought and gained for interested clinical supervisors to participate. There was general consensus that the first meeting would be face-to-face to allow everyone to get to know each other, to set up the process and work out the technology. Six clinicians from two metropolitan services and two regional services came together to form a clinical supervision support group. The aim was to support each other in their roles as clinical supervisors and provide the opportunity for less experienced clinical supervisors to engage with clinical supervisors with broader experience, knowledge and skills. In my experience of facilitating video conferencing supervision for supervisors, there are a number of practical considerations in getting started (Box 7.4), which also include training participants in the use of the technology beforehand.

BOX 7.4	*Some practical considerations when preparing to use video conferencing for clinical supervision*
	■ Gain authority to use the video conferencing facility for clinical supervision ■ Pre-arrange which location is initiating the call and how costs will be managed between the participants ■ Arrange a visit to the video conferencing area and assess the environment for privacy, comfort, booking arrangements and technical support, and arrange a training session

BOX 7.4	(cont'd)

- Develop and circulate a step-by-step process sheet for dialling in or connecting to each area
- Gain an agreement beforehand or in the first session particularly in relation to confidentiality, e.g. documentation, whether the session is to videoed or transcribed
- Set up a group email beforehand so everyone can indicate their intention to attend or not prior to the session to reduce waiting time at the beginning
- At the training session ensure everyone has an opportunity to experiment with the equipment and get some experience of the audio and video quality and requirements for its use
- The event needs to be planned; block booking video conference sessions in advance with a gap allowance of 15 minutes either side of your session increases the availability of time slots. Each area will then need to make corresponding arrangements.
- Ensure that telephone communication is available in all locations in case of connection problems
- Arrange to meet early for the first meeting and run through the process
- Start the session connection at the pre-arranged time — don't wait for stragglers or other locations won't know what is happening
- Agreement on the structure of the session, including timing, is important; the usual length of the session is around one hour to maintain concentration
- Although a learning experience, having someone facilitate each area will reduce interruptions and keep the flow of the session
- Decide if the process is to be supported in other ways; i.e. occasional face-to-face meetings, telephone or online.

The process for conducting the video conferencing supervision sessions for supervisors was:

- Facilitator welcomes group members
- Facilitator appoints a time keeper
- Supervisee(s) brings issue(s) to discuss in the session and works with the peer supervisors
- 5–10 minutes were allocated to summarize the session
- Each participant provided verbal feedback on what they liked 'best' and 'least' about the session and evaluating ways of improving the method
- Participants kept their own supervisory notes and reflections
- Each session was finished on time

Our evaluation of the video conferencing clinical supervision process indicated a high commitment to the initiative evidenced by the regular turnout for each of the sessions. Specifically, our experience of using video conferencing technology as group supervisors in clinical supervision revealed that:

- The video conferencing audio and video quality was of a high quality and caused minor delays and was well sequenced

BOX 7.4	(cont'd)

- Minor technical hitches such as the 'mute' button being on and the occasional need for screen and volume adjustment
- No problems were encountered with connections due to the development and publication of a step-by-step process sheet
- Participants reported a strange experience they encountered immediately post video conferencing sessions. Although they had finished the session with the whole group they would have further discussion with the smaller group, giving a sense of being part of two groups. This was not seen as a negative thing but worth reporting
- Waiting for permission to talk was problematic initially, but overcome with the appointment of a facilitator at each location
- The use of body language, hand movements or leaning forward indicated a person's intention to speak
- It was noticed that there was a tendency to focus on the people on the screen and to some extent provide little on no eye contact with other people at the same location
- Facilitators were challenged when 1:1 monologue discussions started to emerge in the session, taking up the 'air time' and reducing the participation and effectiveness of the group

Each session cost AUD $90 or around £45 GBP for one hour, which was considered cost-efficient compared to the cost of travel if face-to-face clinical supervision had been adopted. Group participants generally reported finding that the session structure and its content distracted them from focusing on the technology (everyone expressed satisfaction with this technology). A face-to-face evaluative session was arranged after the process had been in operation for 6 months. Although it was expected that we would be discussing the benefits and burdens of video conferencing technology it was interesting to find that very little time was spent on this. Rather, the group briefly mentioned some of the things they had learnt about the technology in a positive way and quickly moved on to discussing their own thoughts and feelings of the clinical supervision support group process. Individuals commented on how valuable they had found the sessions for reflecting on their own personal advancements in knowledge, skill and know how. The group reflected back on when the sessions commenced and stated how quickly the group seemed to bond and individually how safe they felt; for instance one participant commented:

> … It felt safer than doing clinical supervision with colleagues in my own workplace, I felt less inhibited in discussing some of those more difficult issues and it was easier to challenge others …

Normalizing the things that occurred in the video conferencing clinical supervision process was highlighted as being extremely important to individual supervisors. The video conferencing supervisors' group unanimously decided to continue and attempt to replicate this process for others within their organizations. Our experience of video conferencing technology for clinical supervision in remote areas is viewed as a 'means to an end'. As with any information and communication technology being utilized for clinical supervision purposes, while potential barriers need to be acknowledged, there are very likely to be associated benefits to support the process.

ISSUES IN ONLINE AND TEXT-BASED CLINICAL SUPERVISION

With the advance of computers and online networks — especially the internet — a further dimension of human experience is rapidly opening up. Although the technologies are different, real-time online interaction via the internet is not dissimilar to telephone and video conferencing technologies, outlined previously, with similar advantages and disadvantages. We wonder how many of you when 'logging on' to your online service, launching a programme, or about to compose an email feel — consciously or subconsciously —that you are entering in, or travelling to, a remote 'space' often referred to as 'cyberspace'. Computer language promotes this idea by using words such as 'domains' or 'rooms'. Suler (1999) offers an excellent, constantly updated hypertext book examining the psychology of cyberspace. Could such ideas be extended to clinical supervision in that you go to 'another place for space', with someone you might not know that well, to 'talk' in cyberspace about your world of practice?

While it is probably not yet usual in your own clinical supervision, exploring the frontiers of online or text-based technology in counselling and mental health arenas is expanding. For instance, the Australian Psychological Society (APS 2005) estimate that there are over 500 telephone and internet-based 'services' offering a combination of information, support and counselling; they are playing a major role in the provision of health and community welfare and they are likely to increase by approximately 20 to 30 per cent per year. The International Society for Mental Health Online (ISMHO), a non-profit organization formed in 1997, actively seeks to promote the understanding, use and development of online communication, and information technology for the international mental health community. The ISMHO has published guidelines for those engaged in online therapeutic work (ISMHO 2000), and a detailed paper outlining some of the myths and realities of online work (Fenichel et al 2002) when compared to face-to-face encounters. Finally, in the UK, the Samaritans, a volunteer-based telephone help organization, has extended its telephone service and now receives and responds to over 1,750 emails each week (Samaritans 2005).

One of the obvious advantages of increased technology becoming available in online or text-based counselling and therapy is that the provision of services is increasingly becoming more flexible and accessible. It also facilitates a client's ability to choose when and how those services are used and challenges the assumption that it is even necessary to meet in a therapist's office to gain benefits as a service user. While the internet and text-based technology is cited as being useful in a therapy setting, how possible might it be to transfer online principles into your own clinical supervision situation? How might those same online principles in the therapy setting be similar or dissimilar?

Perhaps, unlike unfamiliar video conferencing technology, the familiarity of using the internet or 'going online' from the comfort of your own home might have greater or lesser appeal to those unable to gain access to a clinical supervisor in their organization. After all, it only took a chance email for Allan and myself to begin networking across continents and then to physically meet up and work with each other. The rest as they say is history!

… in 1985 the internet connected a mere 2000 computers, by the turn of the century it connected 30 million … by 2005 it is projected there will be more than one billion computer users …
Armstrong and Schneiders, 2003:129

It is extremely likely that you, like us, are one of those one billion computer users, allowing the doors of possibility to swing open for those currently working in practice without access to clinical supervision. According to Stofle and Hamilton (1998), online supervision could even replace ongoing face-to-face supervision in the social work setting, particularly when the supervisor and supervisee are separated by great distance. However as Fenichel (2003:75) rightly points out, the internet is simply a tool and not the clinical supervision process itself. Although we have both experimented with electronic mail clinical supervision as a supplement to the telephone, online supervision remains in its infancy and is something we have only begun to utilize and we acknowledge our limitations in practising what we preach.

A good place to look specifically for information about the exciting developments in online supervision, whether to become a supervisor, or gain access to clinical supervision yourself, is http://www.online-supervision.net where a major international and multiprofessional evaluation of computer-mediated clinical supervision is underway (Group InterVisual 2003). At the time of writing, John has since applied to join this online group. Another international online group commenced in March 2002 for mental health practitioners and researchers, with an interest or involvement in the practice, research, development or theory of online clinical supervision and psychotherapy, currently offers, after registering, an email list (psychotherapy-online@jiscmail.ac.uk), video conferencing and instant message facility, and website (http://www.psychotherapy-online.net). The forum's function is to exchange theory, experience and research, and offer an opportunity for networking, sharing information, supporting and challenging those practising or researching in these fields. A North American strategic overview, combining online with other available technologies for allied health practitioners involved in clinical supervision (Miller et al 2003), can be accessed along with many other online clinical supervision resources at http://supervisionresource.com. This is in addition to the UK-based clinical supervision resources that can be found at http://clinical-supervision.com and http://supervisionandcoaching.com.

Many of the issues with online and text-based clinical supervision using alternative technology (Table 7.1) have been discussed earlier. However there are specific advantages and disadvantages to consider when using online and text-based technology for clinical supervision and these are summarized in Table 7.2.

You can probably think of many other advantages and disadvantages that have not been included in Table 7.2.

The literature on electronic or email supervision, unlike that on online supervision, remains sparce despite them both having a textual element. Perhaps there is not a need to separate the methods. However, it is worth mentioning

TABLE 7.2 *Some specific advantages and disadvantages when utilizing online and text-based methods for clinical supervision*

Advantages	Disadvantages
Being anonymous can make it easier to express in text language what is being thought or felt at a given time	Difficulties in knowing what 'here and now' really means with differing global time zones and variation in delivery of email communications
Permanent records can be kept of text or email conversations for future reference or for research purposes	The need to have a knowledge of receiving, storing and protecting confidential data
Online and text methods can be optionally supplemented with 'real-time' conversations by telephone or in face-to-face meetings	Online and text language can be open to cultural misinterpretation in the absence of visual clues
Pauses between questions allow for more reflective thinking time	The need to be tolerant with delays in receiving online or text responses
Able to work in the comfort of your own home or office at a time that suits the individual(s)	Working on the computer alone, even in a 'group' situation, can be more isolating than working face-to-face
Wider opportunities for clinical supervision to happen in remote locations	Technical problems such as network speed, adding new software or not being able to connect
Having access to a computer extends the range of clinical supervision opportunities	Difficulties in mastering basic typing skills and slowing down the communication process (particularly synchronous communications)
Increased flexibility for the practitioner with online and (or) email methods of clinical supervision	The need to be adaptable with online relationships (asynchronous/synchronous)
Accumulating body of knowledge online particularly in mental health arenas that can be adapted for clinical supervision	Research activities cannot keep pace with improvements in technology

that a preference for peer group supervision seems evident when working with email (Livingstone 1999, McMahon (undated), Stebnicki & Glover 2001). May (2000) outlines some of the benefits and disadvantages of offering one-to-one email supervision based on his experiences in the UK over a period of one year. His supervisees benefited from having a supervisory structure, including written proformas to work from and guidelines for presenting a case beforehand.

Having both had experience of using this method of clinical supervision in an asynchronous way with each other, we concluded that having a permanent record was an advantage (to measure progress) and that meeting beforehand produced a more relaxed process of communication (because a relationship had been established). However, anonymity can have a disinhibiting effect on participants, who under such circumstances may feel more free to express themselves. While email supervision might be able to 'fill the supervision drought' (McMahon — undated) and it might be an option you consider for yourself, there can be significant stresses with the method (Suler 2003).

Working alone with emails can be a stressful activity! How many do you receive when you open your mailbox? Deciding on an email option as clinical supervision might contribute to feeling overwhelmed with yet more information and things to do!

In this chapter we have exposed you to a number of alternative ways to engage in clinical supervision based on advances in technology. You may have been surprised, as well as confused, by the range of possibilities open to you. The idea that there is not enough time, or there are enough supervisors around to offer clinical supervision, as an argument for not getting started, we would suggest, is wearing a bit thin. While engaging in a face-to-face encounter might be the ideal, for those working in rural or remote areas the utilization of an alternative technology might be the only clinical supervision option.

Reflect on some of the realities of your own work situation with regard to accessing clinical supervision or being in clinical supervision

Review the range of technological options identified in the chapter, perhaps following up some of the referenced websites for using the methods:
- telephone
- video conferencing
- online
- email
- supplementary combinations of either of the above

Write down and discuss with colleagues why some clinical supervision options might be more suitable than others.

Decide on *one* clinical supervision option you wish to take forward as an idea and set out a timeframe for getting started and then do it

Email either of us to let us know what your experiences were

John: admiralpd@btopenworld.com

Allan: allant@bhs.org.au

CONCLUSION

The intention behind this chapter was to outline some of the more common information and communication technologies available for use with getting started with clinical supervision. Much of the current literature and direct experience has been led by health professionals in mental health, counselling and psychotherapy and our challenge to you in other healthcare arenas is to capture what method you intend to use and develop the knowledge with others. It is important that your choices of alternative technological methods of clinical supervision do not present a further barrier to getting started at all. If technological options are not your thing then leave it alone and seek out more traditional face-to-face encounters. However, we continue to be amazed how relatively simple it is to network and gain clinical supervision globally from the comfort of your own sitting room or office!

Finally, you might remember Allan's metaphor derived from his previous background as a worker on the railways ... *you can either drive the train or just be part of the track*! So, while we acknowledge that the face-to-face encounter might currently be the preferred method for healthcare professionals' clinical supervision, we feel that it is unlikely to remain unchallenged as the preferred method for much longer.

On reflection ... chapter summary

- The use of alternative technological methods will support the continued development of clinical supervision, particularly in remote and rural areas of practice
- The use of alternative technological methods will reduce some of the practical barriers often faced in getting started with clinical supervision
- Effective communication and relationship development is still possible even when not meeting in a face-to-face situation
- There is an increased need to consider confidentiality issues and how these will be managed when using alternative technologies in clinical supervision
- The traditional face-to-face clinical supervision encounter is becoming challenged by technological opportunities to access appropriate clinical supervisors across great distance
- With any of the alternative technologies available to use in clinical supervision there will be practical realities to consider beforehand to increase its effectiveness
- The use of alternative technological methods for clinical supervision in mainstream healthcare is still in its infancy, providing further research opportunities

REFERENCES

Anthony K 2003 The use and role of technology in counselling and psychotherapy. In: Goss S, Anthony K (eds) Technology in counselling and psychotherapy: a practitioner's guide. Palgrave, Basingstoke, UK, p 13–34

APS 2005 Telephone and Internet-based Counselling Interest Group (Australian Psychological Society). Online. Available at: http://www.psychology.org.au/units/interest%5Fgroups/tibcp/. Accessed 25/11/05

Armstrong P, Schneiders I 2003 Video and telephone technology in supervision and supervision training. In: Goss S, Anthony K (eds) Technology in counselling and psychotherapy: a practitioner's guide. Palgrave, Basingstoke, UK, p 129–140

Capner M 2000 Video conferencing in the provision of psychological services at a distance. Journal of Telemedicine and Telecare 6:311–319

Cavanagh K, Zack J S, Shapiro D A 2003a The computer plays therapist: the challenges and opportunities of psychotherapeutic software. In: Goss S, Anthony K (eds) Technology in counselling and psychotherapy: a practitioner's guide. Palgrave, Basingstoke, UK, p 165–191

Cavanagh K, Zack J S, Shapiro D A et al 2003b Computer programs for psychotherapy. In: Goss S, Anthony K (eds) Technology in counselling and psychotherapy: a practitioner's guide. Palgrave, Basingstoke, UK, p 143–161

Copeland S 2003 Supervising on the telephone – stop gap solution or effective time management?' Counselling and Psychotherapy Journal (October):34–36

Crago H, Crago M 2002 But you can't get decent supervision in the country. In: McMahon M, Patton W (eds) Supervision in the helping professions. Pearson Education, New South Wales, Australia, p 79–90

Diamond L 1996 Effective video conferencing: techniques for better business meetings. Crisp, Menlo Park, California, USA

Driscoll J, Brown R, Buckley A et al 2006 Exploring the use of telephone group clinical supervision to support the work of practice development nurses in the developing practice network (DPN). Online. Available at: http://www.fons.org/ns/Dissemination_series_reports/DissSeries/vol3No6.pdf/. Accessed 1/7/06

Fenichel M 2003 The supervisory relationship online. In: Goss S, Anthony K (eds) Technology in counselling and psychotherapy: a practitioner's guide. Palgrave, Basingstoke, UK, p 75–92

Fenichel M, Suler J, Barak A et al 2002 Myths and realities of online clinical work – observations on the phenomena of online behavior, experience and therapeutic relationships. A 3rd-year report from ISMHO's Clinical Case Study Group. Online. Available at: http://www.fenichel.com/myths. Accessed 6/12/05

Group InterVisual 2003 An evaluation of computer mediated clinical supervision. The Online Supervision Research Team. Online. Available at: http://www.online-supervision.net/research/protocol1.asp. Accessed 20/12/05

Hadikin R 2004 New to teleclasses – read here first! (teleclass 'etiquette'). Online. Available at: http://www.dreamcoach.co.uk/classes.htm. Accessed 26/11/05

Hogan C 2003 Facilitating distributed teams using technology. In: Hogan C (ed) Practical facilitation a toolkit of techniques. Kogan Page, London, UK, p 377–399

ISMHO 2000 Suggested principles for the online provision of mental health services. International Society for Mental Health Online. Online. Available at: http://www.ismho.org/suggestions.html. Accessed 15 /12/05

Justice T, Jamieson D 1999 The facilitator's fieldbook. American Management Association International, New York, USA

Livingstone A 1999 Professional supervision and support in rural and remote psychology. Conference Paper presented at the South Australian State Psychology Conference (September), Adelaide, South Australia, Telemedicine Publication Resources (Rural and Remote Mental Health Services of South Australia). Online. Available at: http://www.users.bigpond.com/telemed/Publications.htm. Accessed 20/11/05

Mackintosh A 2005 Coaching by telephone? Surely not? The Coaching Manager. http://www.performance-am.com/PDF/Coach%20by%20telephone.pdf. Accessed 25/11/05

Marrow C E, Hollyoake K, Hamer D et al 2002 Clinical supervision using video conferencing technology: a reflective account. Journal of Nursing Management 10:275–282

May A 2000 E-supervision' (distance supervision page). Online. Available at: http://www.adammay.co.uk/distance.htm#telephone. Accessed 12/12/05

McGill I, Beaty L 2002 Action learning – a guide for professional, management and educational development. Kogan Page, London, UK

McMahon M (undated) Structured peer group supervision by email: An option for school guidance and counseling personnel. Online. Available at: http://www.psychology.org.au/units/interest_groups/rural/supervision_email_article.pdf. Accessed 20/12/05

McMahon M, Patton W (eds) 2002 Supervision in the helping professions. Pearson Education, New South Wales, Australia

Miller T W, Miller J M, Burton D et al 2003 Telehealth: a model for clinical supervision in allied health. The Internet Journal of Allied Health Sciences and Practice (July) 1(2). Online. Available at: http://ijahsp.nova.edu/articles/1vol2/MilleretalTelehealth.html. Accessed 15/12/05

Milne D, Oliver V 2000 Flexible formats of clinical supervision: description, evaluation and implementation. Journal of Mental Health 9(3):291–304

Motamedi V 2001 A critical look at the use of video conferencing in United States distance education. Education 122:386–394

Plowman P 2003 Telephone supervision – second class status (Letters). Counselling and Psychotherapy Journal (November):12

Rosenfield M 1997 The counsellor–client relationship. In: Rosenfield M (ed) Counselling by telephone. Sage, London, UK, p 71–101

Rosenfield M 2003 Telephone counselling and psychotherapy in practice. In: Goss S, Anthony K (eds) Technology in counselling and psychotherapy: a practitioner's guide. Palgrave Macmillan, Basingstoke, UK, p 93–108

Samaritans 2005 Questions regarding our email service. Online. Available at: http://www.samaritans.org/talk/email.shtm. Accessed 2/12/05

Sanders P 1996 An incomplete guide to using counselling skills on the telephone. 2nd edn. PCCS Books, Manchester, UK

Simpson S 2003 The use of video conferencing in mental health. Online. Available at: http://www.rcpsych.ac.uk/college/sig/comp/docs/workplace2.pdf. Accessed 19/11/05

Simpson S 2005 Video counseling and psychotherapy in practice. In: Goss S, Anthony K (eds) Technology in counselling and psychotherapy: a practitioner's guide. Palgrave, Basingstoke, UK, p 109–128

Stebnicki M A, Glover N M 2001 E-Supervision as a complementary approach to traditional face-to-face clinical supervision in rehabilitation counselling: problems and solutions. Rehabilitation Education 15:283–293

Stofle G, Hamilton S 1998 On-line supervision for social workers. The New Social Worker 5(4). Online. Available at: http://www.socialworker.com/onlinesu.htm. Accessed 19/12/05

Sturmey R 1994 Clinical supervision by video conferencing in rural and remote areas. The professional effectiveness of video conferencing for supervision. University of New England, Armidale, NSW, Australia, p 15–20

Suler J 1999 Cyberspace as psychological space. Online. Available at: http://www.rider.edu/~suler/psycyber/psychspace.html. Accessed 27/11/05

Suler J 2003 Email communication and relationships. Online. Available at: http://www.rider.edu/%7Esuler/psycyber/emailrel.html. Accessed 27/11/05

Thompson S, Winter R 2003 A telephone-led clinical supervision pilot for nurses in different settings. Professional Nurse 18(8):467–470

Topps D 2005 Did everybody get that? The challenges of international video conferencing. Rural and Remote Health (The International Electronic Journal of Rural and Remote Health Research, Education, Practice and Policy) 5:352. Online. Available at: http://rrh.deakin.edu.au. Accessed 15/11/05

8 Adventures in facilitating group clinical supervision in practice

John Driscoll

INTRODUCTION

The metaphor in the title of the chapter of having an 'adventure' in group supervision, or any form of clinical supervision for that matter, is intended to evoke the idea in (or perhaps even give permission to) health professionals that participating in group supervision can enable collaborative explorations of practice, an opportunity for treading new paths, as well as the likelihood of experiencing some surprises during the process of the group clinical supervision journey. Many of the ideas for this chapter stem from my own experiences of being a supervisee in group supervision, as well as being a facilitator of groups that included group supervision. As a non-therapist, I refer to the term 'facilitator' (of learning) throughout the chapter as opposed to group supervisor, although the terms do seem to be interchangeable in the clinical supervision literature.

On the surface, the potential for collaboratively working in a group way in clinical supervision would seem to be entirely appropriate to consider in the wider organizational sense, given the current healthcare climate for change and reform. However it is worth reflecting on the implications of legitimizing the development of groups in practice that are likely to be microcosms of the wider organization, particularly with the development of multiprofessional clinical supervision groups (Hyrkas & Appelqvist-Schmlechner 2003, Mullarkey et al 2001). It is highly likely and even 'normal' to expect conflicts and uncertainties to emerge as part of the process of having regular and formalized group discussions that are intended to improve practice. The outcomes of such discussions may present even more conflict as health professionals either enable improvements or become disabled by the attempts of individuals determined to maintain the *status quo* — individuals who only appear to rather than actively support the principles of group clinical supervision. For instance, while health professionals, if given the opportunity, would like to implement group supervision as a highly valued method (Butterworth et al 1997), heavy workloads, busy schedules and staff shortages frequently mean that the activity is often not given organizational priority (Hyrkas et al 2002, Sellars 2004, Walsh et al 2003). It requires not only commitment but also creativity to ensure that the development of group supervision activities and approaches are not disrupted.

I am particularly mindful that, for some, the idea of working in a group way can conjure up notions of a being in a form of 'pseudo-therapy' (Yegdich 1999) in unskilled or inexperienced hands. Perhaps this is not surprising as much of the UK clinical supervision literature in the health professions has been, and continues to be, influenced by counselling and psychotherapy frameworks. An obvious difference, to me, between group supervision and therapy is that in the former the focus of concern is usually external to the individual (e.g. clinical practice) and in the latter it is internal to the individual (e.g. personality, relieving symptoms). Therefore, I would suggest for those new to group working that the emphasis be on the health professionals' work and primarily the 'here and now' but with prominence also given to 'future' practice(s). Perhaps much easier to say than do!

In tandem with this are questions raised about the 'appropriateness' (Malin 2000, Rudd & Wolsey 1997) of utilizing therapy-orientated approaches for clinical supervision in acute healthcare environments. A belief that they are inappropriate may also pose a barrier to 'getting started'.

In this chapter, while accepting that there are numerous other approaches that can be adapted for group clinical supervision, I will focus on action learning, Balint and peer group working as workable alternatives to the perceived inappropriate models found in psychological literature. That said, the knowledge derived from psychological research is invaluable; here I have used examples from psychological literature to outline stages of group development and facilitator styles, and Graham Sloan in his chapter discusses the dynamics of groups from a psychological perspective, suggesting that understanding group behaviour might enable the aquisition of protective mechanisms by those feeling vulnerable because they are new to, or are considering setting up, a group situation in practice.

WORKING IN A GROUP WAY TOWARDS CLINICAL SUPERVISION

It might seem strange to even consider working in a group way in clinical supervision when all of you reading this will already have had experience of group working in one way or another, in your personal as well as work lives. But this is the nature of improving practice through reflective practice (described in an earlier chapter); intentionally looking more critically at your routine and taken-for-granted activities can ultimately transform them. I would not be surprised to find that, based on your experiences, you already have some ideas about what might constitute effective and not so effective group clinical supervision and this will ultimately affect your decision to become engaged in the process (or not).

Think about yourself as being a member of two groups … either at work or in your personal life … one group in which you experience personal satisfaction and another in which you might be struggling and would possibly like to leave:
- What, for you, are the key factors in deciding whether or not you like those two groups?
- What are likely to be some of the differences between:
  a) your own behaviour in each of the two groups?
  b) other people's behaviours towards you in each of the groups?
  c) ways that the two groups are managed?

Perhaps some of your ideas about an effective group might have centred on things like members of the group being clear about what is supposed to happen in the group and having some idea of roles and responsibilities, the atmosphere being relaxed, the group being one in which everyone was able to express an opinion and one in which you felt personally valued. On the other hand, you might see an ineffective group as one over-dominated by certain members' opinions, where disagreements make you feel uncomfortable and, because of its poor structure, in which very little seems to be achieved.

Having, as well as expressing, an idea of what some of your hopes, fears and expectations of working in groups are is an essential part of establishing agreement in a clinical supervision group and is discussed in more detail later in the chapter.

I suspect that even if we were able to just get ten readers' responses to the above exercise in their group situations we would be likely to find that:

- their own world views and experiences of working in groups were different;

- each might initially consider their own views as being right for taking forward into the development of group clinical supervision.

Of course, if, in those groups you previously thought about, a spirit of collaboration was encouraged and there was a willingness to arrive at mutually agreed outcomes for group working, despite different points of view, people would be more likely to go away satisfied that their point of view had at least been taken into consideration. However, there are likely to be times when the spirit is unwilling and the need to be right and the need for everyone else to agree that you are right will get in the way of achieving any outcome at all. While diversity in opinion should be welcomed as a source of strength in a group, it can be a challenge to deal with! Alternatively, both of the rather polarized scenarios outlined above, while seeming to present stark differences in group behaviours that may or may not have directly affected you, might also be indicators of quite 'normal' stages in the development of working in groups (rather than being anything sinister).

Numerous models for stages of group development exist, but probably one of the best known and easily understood is by Bruce Tuckman (1965) — revised with Mary Ann Jensen (Tuckman & Jensen 1977). The work was based on looking at the behaviour of small groups and recognizing they went through distinct phases over their lifetimes (Figure 8.1). It has also become part of a web-based working guide for modernizing UK healthcare (NHS Modernization Agency 2006).

In relation to clinical supervision, being aware of the different stages of group development is useful not only to a facilitator but also to the participants who can see whether they are realizing their expected potential or not.

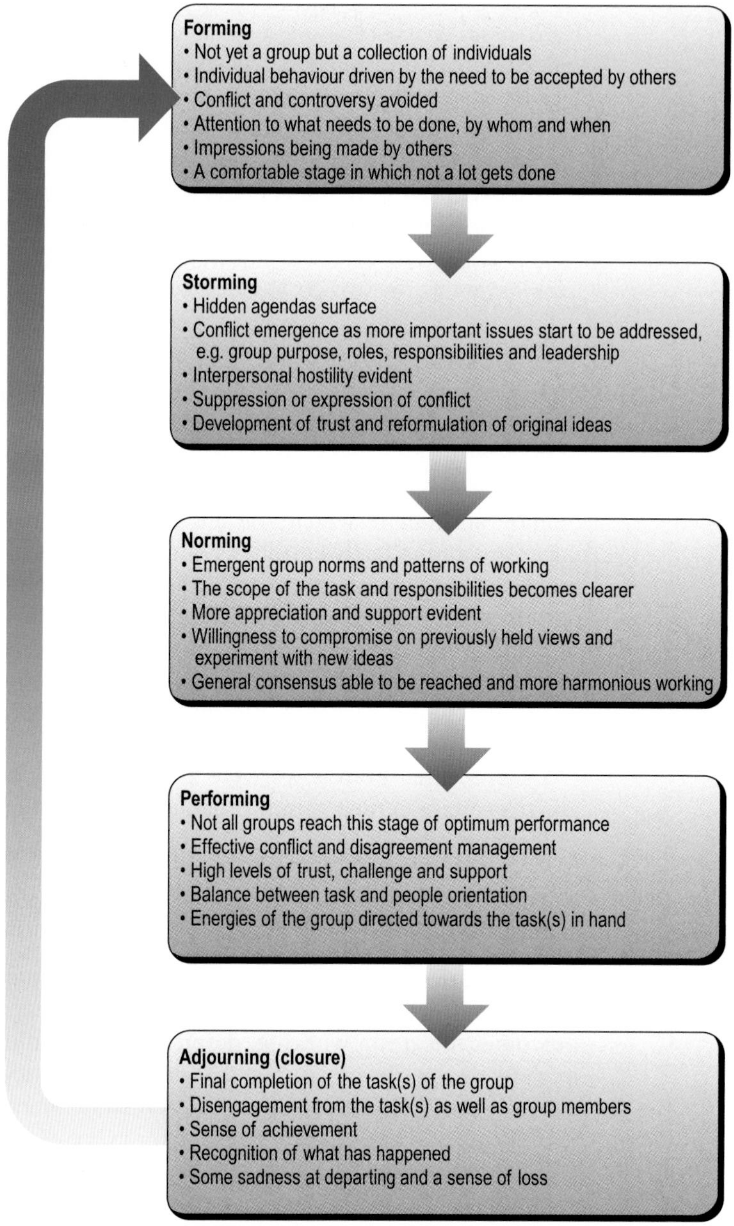

Forming
- Not yet a group but a collection of individuals
- Individual behaviour driven by the need to be accepted by others
- Conflict and controversy avoided
- Attention to what needs to be done, by whom and when
- Impressions being made by others
- A comfortable stage in which not a lot gets done

Storming
- Hidden agendas surface
- Conflict emergence as more important issues start to be addressed, e.g. group purpose, roles, responsibilities and leadership
- Interpersonal hostility evident
- Suppression or expression of conflict
- Development of trust and reformulation of original ideas

Norming
- Emergent group norms and patterns of working
- The scope of the task and responsibilities becomes clearer
- More appreciation and support evident
- Willingness to compromise on previously held views and experiment with new ideas
- General consensus able to be reached and more harmonious working

Performing
- Not all groups reach this stage of optimum performance
- Effective conflict and disagreement management
- High levels of trust, challenge and support
- Balance between task and people orientation
- Energies of the group directed towards the task(s) in hand

Adjourning (closure)
- Final completion of the task(s) of the group
- Disengagement from the task(s) as well as group members
- Sense of achievement
- Recognition of what has happened
- Some sadness at departing and a sense of loss

Figure 8.1 Stages of group development based on Tuckman & Jensen (1977)

Like a living organism, a group will necessarily change and reform and shift into a different developmental stage; e.g. a group that is happily Norming or Performing might move to a different stage of development by the addition (or loss) of participants. It is not always what happens to a group but the way that the 'happening' is dealt with by the group that gives a clue to its stage of development.

A metaphor for capturing the different stages of group life, which I often use, is described by Christine Hogan (2003:99). She depicts the stages of group life as not being dissimilar to the four seasons:

- Winter (the stage of defensiveness),
- Spring (the stage of working through defensiveness),
- Summer (the stage of authentic behaviour),
- Autumn (closure).

The implication for any model you choose to use (if indeed you do) is that the stage the group is in influences other stages, and, in particular, the group's ability to perform to its maximum potential. It also seems useful, as either a participant or facilitator, to have a working knowledge of the different stages of group development, as any individual or group interventions will need to take into account the level of group functioning based on its stage of development.

So, in summary, to understand the complexities of the functioning of any group, it is helpful to have an awareness of:

- the developmental stages of group life,
- the process (the emotional feelings and experiences), and
- the purpose or tasks of the group.

Thinking again about your previous and current involvement in groups, e.g. at work and in educational settings, there will be many benefits as well a number of challenges to consider for undertaking working in a group way in clinical supervision. You might wish to compare your ideas with the contents of Table 8.1.

TABLE 8.1 *Some benefits and challenges for working in a group way at work or in the educational setting*

Benefits of working in a group way	Challenges of working in a group way
A diversity of opinion can be expressed	Issues or concerns raised can seem to go off at a tangent and lack focus
Feelings of an increased sense of support by realizing others have similar concerns	Not everyone will be suited to working in a group way, e.g. feelings of vulnerability
Listening to others concerns can be personally valuable in your own situation	Individual feelings of pressure to conform to a particular way of thinking and not 'rock the boat'
More transparency about what happens in a group	Inner conflicts or feelings can be masked and not addressed
An additional way of personally learning and developing through sharing experiences	Concerns about where individual issues raised might go after the group ends
More cost-effective in time and resources to get things done	Lack of time to deal with an issue or concern in any depth
Able to obtain feedback from others about issues or concerns raised	The dynamics of the group can sometimes make individuals feel uncomfortable
Increased possibilities to share decision-making and responsibilities	The group can sometimes seem to end up as a 'talking shop' with very little being achieved
Being part of a group can lead to deeper friendships being realized	Can be difficult to know everyone and follow through on issues with a fluctuating membership

Having raised some awareness about working in groups generally, it might now become easier to make more informed decisions about the development of your own group clinical supervision in particular.

Working in a group way in clinical supervision, as opposed to self-reflecting on practice, allows practice to be viewed through a 'getting some feedback' lens. The more people in the group, the more potential for feedback! However, too large a group could have drawbacks. Although I interpret 'group' as having at least three participants, the number of participants considered necessary in a group clinical supervision situation remains open to debate. An optimal number seems to rest between five and eight participants, but will be dependent on the amount of time available and the experience of a facilitator/group clinical supervisor.

Despite the challenges posed by group working and the different dynamics that come into play, Butterworth and colleagues (1997) in their national UK study found group clinical supervision to be the preferred option. A number of other authors cite more specific benefits for health professionals becoming engaged in group clinical supervision:

- Reduced professional isolation through increased collaboration between departments (Ashburner et al 2004, Bedward & Daniels 2005).

- A safe environment where health professionals can discuss their limitations and problems without criticism (Dudley & Butterworth 1994).

- A way of containing anxiety through increased self-awareness and professional identity (Arvidsson et al 2001, Jones 2003, Lindahl & Norberg 2002).

- Increased courage to act more confidently and competently in practice (Arvidsson et al 2000, Landmark et al 2004).

- More positive relationships with patients (Severinsson 1995).

- Reduced feelings of stress as more able to manage challenging circumstances in practice (Begat et al 1997, Butterworth 1996, Butterworth et al 1997, Severinsson & Borgenhammar 1997, Williamson & Dodds 1999).

- Increased job satisfaction (Berg et al 1994, Butterworth et al 1997).

- Lower sickness rates (Ashburner et al 2004).

- Retaining the strength and energy to carry on in practice (Arvidsson et al 2001).

- Improved team communication (Hyrkas & Appelqvist-Schmidlechner 2003, Malin 2000).

- A reduction in doubting one's ability to act in practice (Hyrkas et al 2002).

Based on your particular circumstances, you might consider group supervision to be a preferred option (e.g. in terms of the logistics, the prevailing economic conditions and your wish to inspire collaborative working, you may well consider it to be a sensible choice). However, what can present as a solution for one person in the development of clinical supervision in practice, might present as a difficult challenge to another. The clear message is that a choice of suitable clinical supervision formats (e.g. one-to-one situation, group setting) must be available. And keeping in mind that choosing confers a sense of ownership of the thing chosen, choice is a critical factor in the successful implementation of any workable scheme in practice (and described in more detail in the next chapter).

GROUP SUPERVISION APPROACHES

Decisions to commence group clinical supervision will obviously need to be discussed beforehand and it might also be worth dipping into the next chapter on implementing clinical supervision to give you an idea of ways of approaching the matter with staff colleagues. Key questions will be:

- is the group to be an 'open' (fluctuating staff member attendance) or a 'closed' (limited staff membership) group?
- how will the group be organized? and
- what will happen?

Hyrkas and colleagues (2002) describe team supervision as an activity that involves members from differing professional backgrounds but others would refer to this as multiprofessional group supervision as opposed to single professional group supervision (Mullarkey et al 2001). However you refer to it, the group will need to decide what kind of facilitation/supervision should prevail, as there are a number of possibilities:

- Single professional group supervision facilitated by a supervisor from the same discipline, e.g. senior occupational therapist to occupational therapists.
- Single professional group supervision facilitated by a supervisor from a different discipline, e.g. a group of specialist nurses and a counsellor.
- Multiprofessional (team) group supervision facilitated by a designated supervisor, e.g. nominated or a rotating supervisor from within the team.
- Group supervision facilitated by a supervisor external to the organization, e.g. a team of general practitioners from the same practice supervised by a psychotherapist.
- Supervision by professionals from a similar discipline or background or expertise who do not work together on a regular basis, e.g. as part of a regular networking event.

Not all formats of group clinical supervision require the same degree of skill in the processes of group work. There are numerous options for ways of working in groups and more specific attention to psychological approaches in clinical supervision is offered in a previous chapter. Proctor (2000:38), based on the original work of Inskipp and Proctor (1995), suggests four types of group clinical supervision in which the supervisory role can vary from being 'in control' of the process of group supervision, through a continuum of involvement to one where supervisees take responsibility for the process themselves:

- *Authoritative group*: the supervisor is responsible for supervising each participant in turn — supervision *in* a group.

- *Participative group*: The group supervisor is in charge of the supervision but invites other group members to participate and learn how to co-supervise each other — supervision *with* a group.

- *Co-operative group*: Supervisor acts as facilitator for the group with participants sharing and actively involved in the co-supervision of each other — supervision *by* a group.

- *Peer group supervision*: No permanent supervisor, participants share overall responsibility or take turns to be the facilitator.

An example of an authoritative or directive approach to group clinical supervision is when the supervisor (in the truest sense of the word) is a senior manager and there a definite superior–inferior relationship between the supervisor and the supervisees. Examples of this can be found in the UK statutory requirements for child protection supervision (Department of Health 1997) for health visitors and midwives or in managerial forms of group supervision such as caseload supervision in mental health services. While the overriding functions of these forms of group supervision are to monitor, safeguard and protect vulnerable patients or minors, it is questionable whether this is truly group clinical supervision, as it seems there is little emphasis placed by the supervisor on supporting vulnerable health professionals (Davis & Cockayne 2006, Dube undated). A further example of an authoritative group is where supervisees individually reflect on significant practice incidents to the group but remain directed by the supervisor, e.g. a group of junior staff being supervised by a more senior member of staff. Such supervision groups are often characterized by the hierarchical relationship that exists between the supervisor and supervisees and the degree of group control.

Depending on the nature of the group supervision described in the first three types, the role of the supervisee/participant varies between being 'a spectator' (McMahon & Patton 2002:57) of somebody else's supervision in the group, to becoming an active co-supervisor/facilitator. In my experience, it can be useful for those who have never experienced group supervision to have a more structured group supervision experience for an agreed number of meetings. As the group becomes more skilled and builds in confidence, participants/supervisees can then experiment with other types of group supervision, in which the role of the facilitator becomes less overt or directive and participants/supervisees begin to manage their own process. This could be built in as part of the contractual agreement, with regular time for reviewing group skills and shared learning, leading to a self-sustaining group for the future (discussed below).

Intentionally adopting a cascading method in group supervision offers an opportunity for an experiential and work-based learning activity as well as developing ownership of the process. In doing so, the participants/supervisees are able to gradually increase their autonomy and take charge of their own supervision through shared learning, role modelling of group supervisory ideas and experiencing hands-on facilitation. The clear message is around choices being available in clinical supervision whether in a one-to-one situation or the group setting and is a critical factor in the successful implementation of any workable scheme in practice (and described in more detail in the next chapter).

That said, I do agree wholeheartedly with Rolfe et al (2001:102) that the best, perhaps the only, way to learn about group supervision is to actually take part in a group as either a supervisee/participant or a facilitator/participant.

In my experience of facilitating groups to manage themselves in group clinical supervision, it can be helpful, even expected, to offer an initial structure for participants before getting to a stage of what Bernadette, one of my supervisees, referred to as:

> ... being able to ride the horse with your feet, instead of just using the reins ...

While it is beyond the scope of this chapter to go into detail about the very many and varied formats of group clinical supervision, an approach that seems to embrace participative and co-operative formats of group clinical supervision, which might be used as a starting point for a group supervision activity, is a modified form of action learning (McGill & Beaty 2002, RCNI 2000) or the development of action learning groups (Graham 1995, Heidari & Galvin 2003, Platzer 2004).

- Look at the frequently quoted definition of action learning:
  Action learning is a continuous process of learning and reflection that happens with the support of a group or 'set' of colleagues, working on real issues, with the intention of getting things done. The voluntary participants in the group or 'set' learn with and from each other each other and take forward an important issue with the support of the other members of the set.
  McGill & Beaty, 2002:11
- What if the words *action learning* were to be replaced with *clinical supervision*?
- What for you are the key words or ideas that emerge from this definition (if any), in relation to possibilities for your own group clinical supervision?
- What for you would be likely to be a) the task and b) the process if this definition was used for your own group clinical supervision?

While the focus of action learning sets/groups differs according to the situation and the needs of the group as a whole, I would suggest that the general principles would seem to closely align to ideas about group clinical supervision (Box 8.1).

BOX 8.1	*Some principles of action learning that align themselves to group clinical supervision*

- Reflection on real practice issues with the intention of getting things done
- Learning through sharing personal and professional experiences with others
- A combination of challenge and support to change one's situation in practice
- Issues raised based on having a present and future focus
- Dedicated time to be listened to in a safe and confidential environment
- Development of a sense of personal responsibility and commitment to find solutions to and act on questions posed in and by the group
- Dedicated time to review lessons learned with personal progress and group process
- Structures and processes are able to be modified to suit group needs

While, in a group supervision sense, the principles of action learning will tend to focus on individuals within the group, it is most often associated with large project development. In my own experience, I have used action learning principles as a form of group supervision to help implement clinical supervision in organizations. What happens here is that the participants/supervisees in the group contract that the issues or concerns brought to group supervision specifically focus on being related to the implementation of clinical supervision. In this way, a sense of having a shared identity develops in the group (we are all implementing clinical supervision) and group members become 'comrades in clinical supervision adversity' (to adopt the phrase from the founder of action learning, Reg Revans (Revans 1982)). At the same time, by considering other member's experiences, problems or issues about the implementation of clinical supervision, each group member learns from the others in the group.

Although there is no single 'correct' format for action learning, as the process continually evolves over time, there is a commitment, initially by the facilitator, to help individuals work on the tasks presented and avoid becoming embroiled in non-productive general discussions about issues.

Another fundamental function of a group facilitator is the enabling of group independence. The responsibility of running 'set advising' or facilitation should be handed over to the group itself as soon as possible to encourage participants/supervisees to become the owners of their own learning process and subsequent actions.

Other issues to consider in facilitating clinical supervision groups are as follows:

- By having group participants all from the same department there is likely to be a subsequent lack of external perspective — individuals 'not being able to see the wood for trees'

- The number of group participants/supervisees will determine structure (Figure 8.2) and subsequent timings

- The facilitator role in:
  - maintaining a safe environment,
  - keeping a focus on actions,
  - monitoring questioning approaches (in what can often become quite complex issues), and ensuring that a review of the group process occurs

Further information on the principles of action learning can be found in McGill and Beaty (2002), Beaty (2003) and NATPACT (2005).

Acknowledging that 'Action Learning' is a specific approach to management and organizational change and not specifically group clinical supervision:

- What elements of the action learning process might be adapted for group clinical supervision?
- What might be the limitations of adapting action learning principles as group clinical supervision?
- How might the roles of the facilitator be similar to or different from those of the clinical supervisor in the group situation?
- How might the roles of the presenter be similar to or different from those of the clinical supervisee in the group situation?
- What might be some of the advantages and disadvantages of adapting action learning principles as group clinical supervision when:
  a) designing a group where everybody worked with and knew each other?
  b) designing a group where nobody worked with and knew each other?

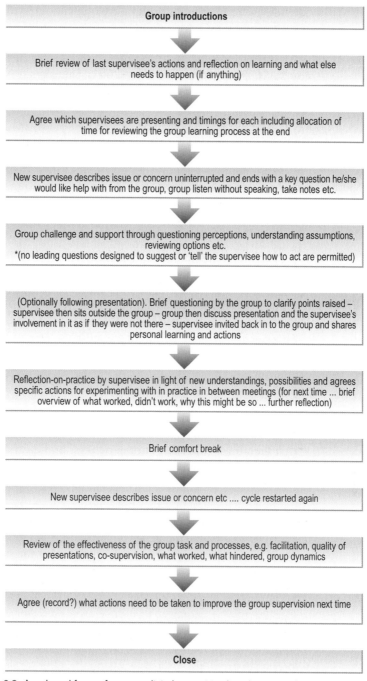

Figure 8.2 An adapted format for group clinical supervision based on action learning meetings

Cottrell and Smith (2000), in their excellent website resource on clinical supervision, propose a different approach to group clinical supervision based on participative co-counselling, where not only is the role of the facilitator prescribed but also a structured approach in getting started is encouraged. They warn that, depending on the stage of group development, applying structured approaches in group clinical supervision might be too restrictive but that rotating roles and building in a review of the process will benefit the leadership of the whole group.

An interesting approach, and one of the earliest methods of clinical supervision for family doctors (Horder 2001, Salinsky 2003), is the Balint Group approach (Balint 2000) established in the 1950s and named after Michael Balint (a psychoanalyst from Hungary). It has since spawned a number of international Balint Societies and websites. Although a Balint leader is trained and accredited in the method, the principles behind the Balint approach might well be applicable in certain group supervision situations. The Balint discussion groups intentionally stimulate family doctors to examine their understandings of the emotional content of the doctor–patient relationship and explore alternative ways of responding (The Balint Society 2006). The closed group discussions, less concerned with finding solutions, focus on exploring relationships (Salinsky 2003:81). The facilitator role is amply described as follows:

> Presentations are spontaneous, based on priority issues from within the group, without the use of notes for around five minutes followed by composition of a key question for the group to consider. After a short period of factual, rather than feeling questions to elicit clarity, the presenter 'pushes back' and takes no further part in the discussion remaining an observer for around 20 minutes whilst the rest of the group discuss the question before then rejoining the group.

The facilitator is mainly concerned with the psychological group processes described by Johnson et al (2004) as:

> ... self reflection and exploration of meaning rather than problem solving is the key to Balint leadership ... it is not the leader's individual brilliance that illuminates the case, but the richness and diversity of the group participation and interactions he/she facilitates ...

My rationale for including what is essentially medical practitioner group supervision into the discussion is that the principles might be applied to those working in more technical areas of clinical practice (such as intensive care, neonatal units, theatres, accident and emergency departments), where, more often than not, the patients are too much in need of (life) support for the staff to then get any!

As a charge nurse in intensive care in a previous life, I would have welcomed the formal support that specialist external supervisors such as mental health practitioners or chaplains might have brought to often distressing situations. As it was, my distress tended to be sorted out informally in a coffee room or over a beer afterwards and somehow just seemed to get buried — but I remember those patients and relatives, including their names, and the remembrance of the associated distress still surfaces occasionally, almost twenty years on. It seems to me that a modified Balint group approach with a supervisory eye firmly fixed on improving relationships with patients (as well as difficult staff) might be protective for both staff and patients.

The final dip into group supervisory approaches involves peer group working. In this approach there is no permanent group facilitator, with the role often being rotated between individual members of the group or members working in pairs (co-facilitation). While seemingly a straightforward option for group clinical supervision with a captured audience to hand, it can be more challenging than at first seems and it can be helpful to have an external or experienced group facilitator to begin the process. In a recent experience, while working as an external consultant to support the development of peer group supervision with senior physiotherapists, who were all of the same grade and experience, I had to pay particular attention to the structure of the meetings and the contract. Aside from the practicalities of finding the space to regularly meet as a peer group, which was challenging, I was interested to observe the behaviours displayed in this peer group supervision; behaviours that were 'normal' in their everyday clinical practice. For instance:

- talking over each other,
- having side conversations,
- not listening,
- interrupting each other's conversations.

And behaviours that reflected their attitude toward being in a clinical supervision group:

- absenteeism and lateness in starting,
- feeling guilty about attending while colleagues worked.

While working in what are sometimes called 'concentric circles' (an inner working supervision group and an outer group of observers), those same taken for granted normal behaviours became glaringly obvious and significant for the observers — it became clear that there was a need for a contract regarding the conduct of the group. This demonstrates how less noticeable things are when there is a familiarity between peers working in the same culture who have developed close relationships. Playle and Mullarkey (1998) cite how the unconscious dynamics of relationships at work can often be mirrored within behaviours displayed in group clinical supervision or what they refer to as 'parallel processing'. A possibility for 'making the unnoticed more noticed', in groups where a closeness exists, is to ensure (as part of the contractual agreement) that time is built into the meetings for reflection on what has happened in the group and the obtaining of sensitive 'observer' feedback — particularly when peer group supervision is a new process in practice.

Turner and colleagues (2005), in the development of peer group supervision as a form of networking supervision for specialist nurses, reported similar behaviours to those I had observed:

> ... at our first attempt to tackle a clinical issue, without prompting or guidance, the group used its usual problem solving approach. Its application in this situation meant we all wanted to talk over each other, offering advice and solutions so that the individual presenting the situation for discussion felt attacked rather than supported. The whole experience was very distressing. Our second attempt, using facilitation and guidance, enabled us to reflect upon this and then approach another scenario using new techniques, which enabled the presenter to reach their own answer/conclusion. This demonstrated a significant change to the group even in that short time.

Considering peer group clinical supervision as an option in and for practice is in itself an invitation to colleagues for increased openness, collaborative working and potential challenge as well as support.

The types and possibilities for working in a group way in clinical supervision are numerous and the working style of any group is likely to alter as the group matures and increases in experience and confidence. But an initial key to any form of working in a group way in clinical supervision is to gain formal agreement on what the group's intentions are and to make sure those intentions are clear to all participants at the outset. A previous chapter by Stephen Power has examined this in more detail, but in groups that are known to have members with conflicting views it is even more important to establish these ground-rules because if potential difficulties are not attended to, disenchantment and even abandonment altogether of the idea of having a group can ensue.

Prior to contracting for group clinical supervision in practice it will be useful to have a meeting with potential group members. You might wish to use the headings contained in Figure 8.3 as a discussion item — or circulate the headings to the group before the first meeting as a form of agenda.

It is extremely unlikely that you will be able to complete all of the items in the first meeting, but it does offer a focus for a discussion. What is important is to get an agreement for how you intend working in group supervision, and this is a useful reference point if at a later stage disagreements begin to surface. Voicing disagreement (as stated earlier in the chapter) is a normal stage of group life and an opportunity to change, rather than necessarily being a negative phenomenon. I would be concerned as a facilitator that the group might be becoming too

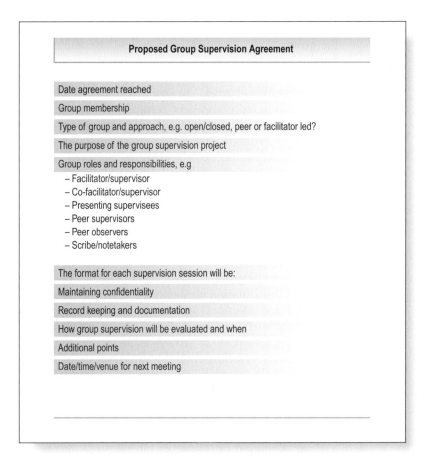

Proposed Group Supervision Agreement

Date agreement reached

Group membership

Type of group and approach, e.g. open/closed, peer or facilitator led?

The purpose of the group supervision project

Group roles and responsibilities, e.g
 – Facilitator/supervisor
 – Co-facilitator/supervisor
 – Presenting supervisees
 – Peer supervisors
 – Peer observers
 – Scribe/notetakers

The format for each supervision session will be:

Maintaining confidentiality

Record keeping and documentation

How group supervision will be evaluated and when

Additional points

Date/time/venue for next meeting

Figure 8.3 Key headings for gaining agreement in the development of group clinical supervision

collusive without some form of positive challenge or dissent! For instance, Walsh et al (2003) in the development of their group supervision decided on the following set of group norms:

■ Commitment to supervision and the group

■ Meetings should start and finish on time

■ All members to attend except where an unforeseen clinical issue places a client at risk

■ Preparedness to disclose and take risks

■ Receptiveness to others' views

■ Responsibility of the presenter to be prepared beforehand

■ Supportive critical friendship attitude

■ Confidentiality with exceptions, e.g. cases where unsafe, unprofessional or potentially dangerous conduct is identified

The role of the facilitator/supervisor is a key aspect of effective group clinical supervision working in which, as we have seen, a number of different approaches can be employed. While it is very likely that a facilitator/supervisor will have had considerable experience in working with groups, some groups might be experimental, rather than experiential, particularly in a peer group situation. Therefore it is useful to get some basic ideas about the challenges and choices when facilitating group supervision for the first time, although this is not a substitute for gaining further training from within your own learning resources (e.g. through independent trainers or from your local education provider). You may already have ideas about this before commencing any group supervision project.

CHALLENGES AND CHOICES WHEN FACILITATING GROUP CLINICAL SUPERVISION

A common advertising slogan is *size matters* and it is certainly worth thinking about when facilitating group supervision. Within groups an absent or new participant can alter the whole group dynamic. For instance, in more structured and participative groups where differing roles are critical to the overall process, absenteeism can make a profound difference to what was intended to happen, as well as leading to concerns being raised about the commitment towards group supervision. Likewise, introducing a new person into the group is likely to alter the group dynamics back to a previous stage of development (Figure 8.1), but might also be an invigorating change to the life and workings of the group. I have known some groups to state, as part of the contracting process, that if a person misses a group on two consecutive occasions, and if apologies are not sent, they cannot return. It is therefore critical to group functioning to discuss such matters on commencing group supervision, including whether the group intends to be 'closed' (fixed membership) or 'open' (dip in and out and mixed membership). Of course, the larger the group the more complex the facilitation becomes.

Johns (2001) wisely warned that, depending on the intent and emphasis of the supervisor, clinical supervision can be a very different experience for supervisees.

What he exposed in his research was how the underlying tensions in individual supervisors' perceptions and organizational ideas about the nature of clinical supervision will impact on the way clinical supervision is organized. This is a key consideration in working in a group way as a clinical supervisor for the first time. Hawkins and Shohet (2002:134) suggest that unless supervisees are already experienced in group work they are very likely to be influenced by the styles of their group supervisors. They outline four quadrants depicting differing styles (Figure 8.4) a group supervisor can move through with supervisees, depending on the needs of the group and the stage of group development.

Clearly it is important for all those involved in decision-making about how group supervision is organized that there is a conscious awareness that alternative group styles exist depending on the stage of group development (Figure 8.1) and the experience of the group as a whole, including the group supervisor. New group supervisors may well need to consider whether their preferred style is an intentional choice, or simply based on their own understandings and experience on what they think group clinical supervision is. I would suggest that the facilitator/supervisor role be an item of discussion right from the start with participants/supervisees when making a contractual agreement (*see* Figure 8.3).

The different styles, far from making choices in the group clinical supervision process even more complex, simply offer a range of opportunities for the group,

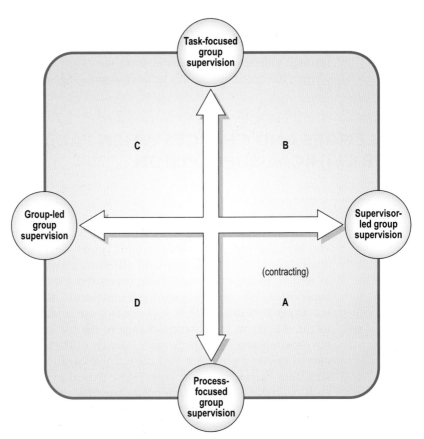

Figure 8.4 Summary of facilitation styles and group structures in clinical supervision based on Hawkins P, Shohet R (2002) Supervision in the helping professions, 2nd edn. Open University Press, McGraw-Hill Education

as well as the intended group supervisor. While acknowledging my own bias for reflective learning in group clinical supervision, the whole process can become a shared, or co-learning, experience and an adventure in itself for the whole group, including the supervisor, provided that there are built-in opportunities for feedback, learning and subsequent improvement.

This section of the chapter is concerned with the facilitation of group clinical supervision in its widest sense; in that a group exists for the purposes of clinical supervision and that the process is overseen by a single group supervisor (facilitator), or rotating group supervisors (facilitators), or directed by the group members themselves. In all formats, I would suggest it is helpful to the group supervisor to have some sort of reference point on which to base facilitation, or as the Latin root of the word means, 'to make it easier' (for the group). Bens (2000:7) likens the role of a facilitator to a match referee:

> … rather than being a player, a facilitator acts more like the referee. That means you watch the action, more than participate in it. You control which activities happen, keep your finger on the pulse of the game and know when to move on or wrap things up …

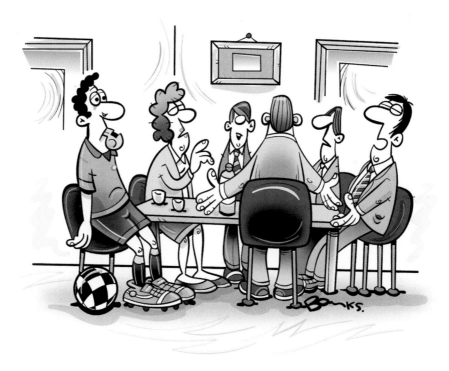

While I recognize that this may be an ideal, where possible, it is easier if the facilitator, like the referee, is non-partisan and detached from the hurly-burly of clinical practice. By not having an emotional attachment to the group in its everyday roles or tasks, it is much easier to observe what the group cannot see and (with permission) raise matters that the group finds difficult. Not long ago I recently facilitated a group of healthcare scientists to set up their own group supervision. Not being emotionally involved and not being very clear about their everyday work allowed me to see and name the 'elephant in the room' (the thing nobody knows quite what to do with because of its enormity and avoids talking about). That elephant was the reorganization of laboratories that had led to acrimonious relationships in the directorate. Once this had been identified it was unable to be ignored and the group focused on how to manage it.

In a group supervision situation the facilitator needs to balance the responsibilities for enabling the group to manage their 'task' with being attentive to the group 'process'. The task of the group supervision (or what's happening) will be quite obvious as this would have been structured and verbally agreed in advance (e.g. two supervisees present their situations in the time allowed, with a time for feedback). The process of the group supervision (how it's happening) relates to what is not being verbalized, is less visible and is associated with the more psychological aspects of the group (such as how the group members seem to relate to each other, the group atmosphere, feelings people are having towards each other). Rogers (2002:7) eloquently summarizes this as:

> ... the task concerns the head and the process concerns the heart ... for effective group working, both the heads and hearts of ... (*group supervisees*) ... will need to be satisfied ...

(The words in italics are mine.)

In reality, the group facilitator's role, skills and attributes lie on a continuum from actively 'doing for others' (assisting the group with their specific tasks and goals) to 'enabling those same others' (through supportive challenge, to developing alternative ways of seeing, learning and subsequently working).

In summary, the three overlapping functions of the facilitator (Figure 8.5) are reminders that the effective facilitation of group supervision is interdependent, will not remain static and is a dynamic and ongoing process.

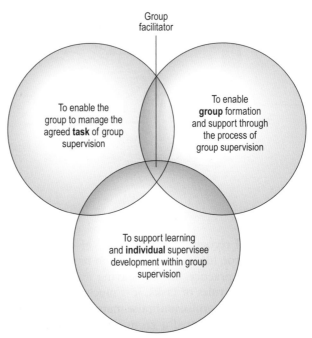

Figure 8.5 The three overlapping functions of the group facilitator in group supervision (based on Adair 1987)

For instance, if the task or intentions of group supervision have not been agreed with the group from the start or not enough attention is being paid to ongoing group processes (which might not be that obvious), not only will the task of group supervision suffer, but also individual supervisees in the group will be dissatisfied. Similarly, if the individual needs of the supervisee are not being met, the group will become ineffective and the purpose of group supervision will struggle to become realized.

Look at the three functions of the group facilitator contained in Figure 8.4 that focus on the:
■ Task needs of the group.
■ Individual needs within the group.
■ The needs of the group as a whole.
　What would you consider your current strengths are within each of those three functions of facilitating groups?
　What functions of group facilitation would you personally find challenging and how might you deal with these?
　What are your likely development needs in facilitating group supervision effectively?
How helpful is this facilitation framework work in describing what might be happening in groups you currently belong to and offering alternative ways of more effective working?

The challenges and choices presented by facilitating really bring home to me, in my work, that learning to become an effective facilitator is a continually ongoing process; this is the very essence of lifelong learning in clinical supervision. This is not really surprising as each group is, in a sense, unique, because of the variability of the skills and personalities of its members, and therefore the facilitator's responses must adapt to this variability. In other words, the facilitator has to learn new ways or adapt old ways to effectively facilitate.

I purposely use the term facilitator to remind me that in whatever group I function in I am a co-learner rather than an experienced supervisor or some sort of expert. It is also useful when the going gets tough for me in a group as a facilitator that I am willing to learn from that group situation and state this to the group (something that is harder to do if you have placed yourself 'in charge' of the group). Peter, a psychotherapist colleague of mine, playfully suggested that my refusal to take on the role of 'expert' in my facilitation of group supervision might be a 'judo move' on my part to avoid conflict. I have pondered this often and accept that there probably is more than a grain of truth in this. I do like to be liked and this continues to present me with a challenge as well as choices … on the other hand perhaps he was only joking? —Yet another example of how I (as a facilitator), continually fail to see things as they are (although I try to in groups), but really see things as I am, hence the need for ongoing supervision to remain effective!

I state this to offer hope to new group facilitators that the work is never done and there is always room for improvement regardless of how much training or experience you have. While I think it is perfectly possible to simply run your own group supervision from scratch, it is only fair to that group that any potential facilitator has an idea of some of the more common challenges and choices posed in group working. Thinking about this, I offer a 12 point survival guide for new group facilitators in Box 8.2.

While the discussion in this chapter has tended to focus on how to get started with group clinical supervision and some thoughts on what to do while it is going on, I think it wise to now consider how to end clinical supervision even though you might just be beginning. While the process of learning as a facilitator is a lifelong adventure, there will be a time when group clinical supervision finally comes to an end or conclusion.

ENDING GROUP CLINICAL SUPERVISION (AND THE CHAPTER!)

As I think it important to consider how to draw group supervision to a conclusion, I was surprised that 275 clinical supervision articles, identified in a literature search by Chambers and Cutcliffe (2001), did not make any specific reference to issues of ending clinical supervision in their titles or key words.

Endings are significant and Chambers and Cutliffe (2001) acknowledge this when they comment that as working in groups involves an investment in time, commitment and energy it can be with some sadness as well as some joy that the work comes to an end.

BOX 8.2	*A 12 point survival guide for new facilitators of group supervision*

1. Find out how others have facilitated groups before starting, e.g. networking with colleagues, educators, literature searching, surfing the web

2. Sort out some clinical supervision for yourself with somebody who has some experience of group working.

3. Have a basic structure in your mind for the duration of the group.

4. Prepare a list of open questions that you can refer to.

5. Start small and gain some confidence in group working.

6. Consider a co-facilitator role but be clear about who is doing what.

7. Get agreement with the group on some basic group rules as well as what is intended to happen.

8. Get as many people actively involved in the process and rotate roles to see what others do, e.g. observers, scribe, timekeeper, supervisees

9. Listen more than you say.

10. Promote silence and space to think.

11. Observe what is happening in the group, rather than your impressions of what is being said by supervisees.

12. Allow time for feeding back on the whole process, including being open to how you did.

What sorts of experiences have you had with relationships coming to an end at work?

For example:

- a colleague leaves the department,
- completion of a course of study,
- a lengthy project you had been involved in comes to an end,
- a regular meeting comes to an end.

What sorts of feelings did it leave you with?

How might this affect your reactions to group clinical supervision coming to an end or even beginning?

Power (1999:205) cites three main reasons why clinical supervision groups might close before the work is completed:

- causes not connected to the supervisory relationship,
- a breakdown in the supervisory relationship,
- the sudden termination of the supervisory relationship.

For most clinical supervision groups I work with, for contractual reasons, there is an intended end-point set at the beginning — normally at the end of anything from six to ten sessions. I am often employed to get things started and furnish the group with the necessary tools for it to continue once I leave. In these cases, the ending is planned for as well as expected and the closing ceremony (usually with some cakes and coffee) often centres on formally reviewing achievements and deciding on what then needs to happen. At these ceremonies I often experience mixed emotions: relief that it has finished, a sense of satisfaction at the achievements made, and some sadness at having to say goodbye at that metaphorical station as the train continues on its journey without me. I am sure many group members must also experience mixed emotions tinged, perhaps, with apprehension — what is around the corner?

Sometimes participants in group clinical supervision leave the group because of a change of roles, e.g. promotion or a change in domestic circumstances. At such times acknowledgement must be given to the need of the individual and the group to say their goodbyes and prepare for change.

However, sometimes this is not possible. Turner et al (2005) recount how a group supervisor needed to leave suddenly because of illness:

> After 14 months of supervision ... Having thought we had reached a stage of independence from the supervisor, it was interesting and illuminating to realise this was not the case at all. In our first session 'alone', the old business like approach was again adopted, highlighting the tendency of the group, despite our best intentions, to go back to its old, safe comfortable way of operating ...

It is possible that in times of change, a group, like individuals, might regress back to a stage where it found comfort. However, if the group can perceive this regression, it might strengthen its powers of self-analysis and inspire a determination to move forward once more.

A group can terminate before its intended ending because of a breakdown in relationships, either between the members themselves or between the members and their supervisor. Breakdowns in the supervisory relationship are, thankfully, rare in my experience. They can be due to unresolved personality clashes or power struggles in the group, breaks in confidentiality or feelings of insecurity.

The reason why supervisory relationship breakdowns are rare in groups is that the relationary process is often more transparent (being observed by several eyes) and therefore any possible trouble is identified before it leads to anything serious. Having a working agreement that is regularly reviewed, perhaps in the light of conflict, is an important consideration. If the group does break suddenly there is likely to be animosity and blame appointing but, even worse, the resulting damage may provoke a determination to never participate in group supervision again.

As discussed above, where possible it is important to mark the end of a group and, aside from group reviewing activities, I encourage groups to formally say goodbye. I have found it a nice idea to end with some sort of ceremony (in addition to handing in the standard evaluation forms). A technique I have used is to get participants to draw or sketch a parting gift for each person in the group (including the facilitator). These drawings are then formally presented to each participant to take forward into the future. We end by saying goodbye to each other.

This chapter, as the title suggested, has also been an adventure for me in sharing with you what I consider to be some key ideas for setting up your own group clinical supervision in practice while at the same time promoting collaborative working.

On reflection ... chapter summary

- One of the best ways to learn about facilitating group clinical supervision is to become involved in a group yourself.
- Conflict in group clinical supervision can often lead to change(s) and might also be indicative of the stage of development of the group.
- Effective group clinical supervision working involves attending to group processes as well as the overall task of the supervision.
- Not all formats of group clinical supervision require the same degree of skill in group processes.
- The role of the facilitator in group clinical supervision will be dependent on the approach agreed by the group and may change over time.
- More effective facilitation of group clinical supervision is where the facilitator is also in clinical supervision themself.

REFERENCES

Adair J 1987 Effective teambuilding. Pan, London, UK

Arvidsson B, Lofgren H, Fridlund B 2000 Psychiatric nurses' conceptions of how group supervision in nursing care influences their professional competence. Journal of Nursing Management 8:175–185

Arvidsson B, Lofgren H, Fridlund B 2001 Psychiatric nurses' conceptions of how group supervision in nursing care influences their professional competence: a 4-year follow up study. Journal of Nursing Management 9:161–171

Ashburner C, Meyer J, Cotter A et al 2004 Seeing things differently: evaluating psychodynamically informed clinical supervision for general hospital nurses. Nursing Times Research 9(1):38–49

Balint M 2000 The doctor, his patient and the illness. Churchill Livingstone, Edinburgh, UK

Beaty L 2003 Continuing professional development series (1) action learning. (LTSN Generic Centre) Learning and Teaching Support Network, York, UK. Online. Available at: http://www.heacademy.ac.uk/resources.asp ?process=full_record&section=generic&id =291. Accessed 24/1/06

Bedward J, Daniels H 2005 Collaborative solutions – clinical supervision and teacher support teams: reducing professional isolation through effective peer support. Learning in Health & Social Care 4(2):53

Begat I, Severinsson E, Berggren I 1997 Implementation of clinical supervision in a medical department: nurses' views of the effects. Journal of Clinical Nursing 6:389–394

Bens I 2000 Understanding facilitation. In: Facilitating with ease. Jossey-Bass, San Francisco, CA, USA, p 7–38

Berg A, Hansson U, Hallberg I 1994 Nurses' creativity, tedium and burnout during 1 year of clinical supervision and implementation of individually planned nursing care: comparisons between a ward for severely demented patients and a similar control ward. Journal of Advanced Nursing 20:742–749

Butterworth T 1996 Primary attempts at research-based evaluation of clinical supervision. Nursing Times Research 3(2):151–152

Butterworth T, Carson J, White E et al 1997 It is good to talk. An evaluation study in England and Scotland. University of Manchester, Manchester, UK

Chambers M, Cutcliffe J 2001 The dynamics of 'ending' in clinical supervision. British Journal of Nursing 10(21):1403–1411

Cottrell S, Smith G 2000 A proposed structure for group supervision. Online. Available at: http://www.clinical-supervision.com/ structured%20group%20supervision%20 model.htm. Accessed 20/2/06

Davis G, Cockayne D 2006 Peer support in child protection practice. Journal of Clinical Nursing 20(2). Online. Available at: http://www.jcn.co.uk/ journal.asp?MonthNum=10&YearNum=2 005&ArticleID=856. Accessed 20/02/06

Department of Health 1997 Child protection. guidance for senior nurses, health visitors and midwives and their managers (report of the Standing Nursing and Midwifery Advisory Committee). DOH, The Stationery Office, London, UK

Dube R (undated) Guidance: caseload management for community mental health nurses. Community Mental Health Nurses Association (CMHN). Online. Available at: http://www.amicus-mhna.org/ guidecaseloadmgt.htm. Accessed 10/02/06

Dudley M, Butterworth T 1994 The cost and some benefits of clinical supervision: an initial exploration. International Journal of Psychiatric Nursing Research 1(2):34–36

Graham I 1995 Reflective practice: using the action learning group mechanism. Nurse Education Today 15:28–32

Hawkins P, Shohet R 2002 Group, team and peer-group supervision. In: Hawkins P, Shohet R (eds) Supervision in the helping professions. 2nd edn. Open University, Buckingham, UK, p 127–142

Heidari F, Galvin K 2003 Action learning groups: can they help students develop their knowledge and skills?' Nurse Education in Practice 3:49–55

Hogan C 2003 Practical facilitation: a toolkit of techniques. Kogan Page, London, UK

Horder J 2001 The first Balint group. British Journal of General Practice 51:1038–1039

Hyrkas K, Appelqvist-Schmlechner K 2003 Team supervision in multiprofessional teams: team members' descriptions of the effects as highlighted by group interviews. Journal of Clinical Nursing 12:188–197

Hyrkas K, Appelqvist-Schmlechner K, Paunonen-Ilmonen M 2002 Expert supervisors' views of clinical supervision: a study of factors promoting and inhibiting the achievements of multiprofessional team supervision. Journal of Advanced Nursing 38(4):387–397

Inskipp F, Proctor B 1995 The arts, crafts and tasks of counselling supervision part 1: making the most of supervision. Cascade, Middlesex, London, UK

Johns C 2001 Depending on the intent and emphasis of the supervisor, clinical supervision can be a different experience. Journal of Nursing Management 9:139–145

Johnson A, Nease D, Milberg L et al 2004 Essential characteristics of effective Balint group leadership. Family Medicine 36(4):253–259

Jones A 2003 Some benefits experienced by hospice nurses from group clinical supervision. European Journal of Cancer Care 12:224–232

Landmark B, Wahl A, Bohler A 2004 Group supervision to support competency development in palliative care in Norway. International Journal of Palliative Nursing 10(11): 542–548

Lindahl B, Norberg A 2002 Clinical group supervision in an intensive care unit: a space for relief, and for sharing emotions and experiences of care. Journal of Clinical Nursing 11:809–818

Malin N 2000 Evaluating clinical supervision in community homes and teams serving adults with learning disabilities. Journal of Advanced Nursing 31(3):548–557

McGill I, Beaty L 2002 Action learning: a guide for professional, management and educational development. 2nd edn. Kogan Page, London, UK

McMahon M, Patton W 2002 Group supervision: a delicate balancing act. In: McMahon M, Patton W (eds) Supervision in the helping professions. Pearson Education, New South Wales, Australia, p 55–65

Mullarkey K, Keeley P, Playle J 2001 Multiprofessional clinical supervision: challenges for mental health nurses. Journal of Psychiatric and Mental Health Nursing 8:205–211

NATPACT 2005 Welcome to action learning – archived website of the National Primary and Care Trust Development Programme (NATPACT) part of the NHS Modernization Agency. Online. Available at: http://www.natpact.nhs.uk/ cms/274.php. Accessed 14/2/06

NHS Modernization Agency 2006 General improvement skills (series 3) working with groups. Online. Available at: http://www.wise.nhs.uk/cmsWISE/ Tools+and+Techniques/ILG/ILG.htm or at: www.modern.nhs.uk/improvementguides. Accessed 17/2/06

NHSIA 2001 Action learning: a resource book for Regional Learning Network members (2001-IA-522). National Health Service Information Authority, Leeds, UK

Platzer H 2004 Are you sitting uncomfortably? From group resistance to group reflection in several uneasy moves. In: Bulman C, Schutz S (eds) Reflective practice in nursing. 3rd edn. Blackwell, Oxford, UK

Playle J, Mullarkey K 1998 Parallel process in clinical supervision: enhancing learning and providing support. Nurse Education Today 18(7):558–566

Power S 1999 Groupwork and endings in clinical supervision. In: Power S (ed) Nursing supervision: a guide for clinical practice. Sage, London, UK, p 197–213

Proctor B 2000 A typology for supervision groups. In: Proctor B (ed) Group supervision: a guide to creative practice. Sage, London, UK, p 37–56

RCNI 2000 Realising clinical effectiveness and clinical governance through clinical supervision (a distance learning pack). Royal College of Nursing Institute, Radcliffe Medical, Oxon, UK

Revans R W 1982 The origins and growth of action learning. Chartwell-Bratt, Bromley, Kent, UK

Rogers J 2002 . Introduction. Facilitating groups management futures. London, UK, p 1–8

Rolfe G, Freshwater D, Jasper M 2001 Group supervision. In: Rolfe G, Freshwater D, Jasper M (eds) Critical reflection for nursing and the helping professions. Palgrave, Basingstoke, UK, p 99–126

Rudd L, Wolsey P 1997 Clinical supervision: a hornets nest? Or honey pot? Nursing Times 93(44):25

Salinsky J 2003 Balint groups and the Balint method. In: Burton J, Launer J (eds) Supervision and support in primary care. Radcliffe Medical, Abingdon, UK p 79–90

Sellars J 2004 Learning from contemporary practice: an exploration of clinical supervision in physiotherapy. Learning in Health and Social Care 3(2):64–82

Severinsson E 1995 The phenomenon of clinical supervision in psychiatric health care. Journal of Psychiatric and Mental Health Nursing 2:301–309

Severinsson E, Borgenhammar E 1997 Expert views on clinical supervision: a study based on interviews. Journal of Nursing Management 5:175–183

The Balint (British) Society 2006 Home page – welcome. Online. Available at: http://www.balint.co.uk/. Accessed 28/2/06

Tuckman B 1965 Developmental sequence in small groups. Psychological Bulletin 63(6):384–399

Tuckman B, Jensen N 1977 Stages of small group development revisited. Group and Organizational Studies 2:419–427

Turner K, Laut S, Kempster J et al 2005 Group clinical supervision: supporting neurology clinical nurse specialists in practice. Journal of Community Nursing Online 19(9). Online. Available at: http://www.jcn.co.uk/ journal.asp?MonthNum=09&YearNum=2 005&Type=search&ArticleID=838. Accessed 20/2/06

Walsh K, Nicholson J, Keough C et al 2003
Development of a group model of clinical
supervision to meet the needs of a
community mental health nursing team.
International Journal of Nursing Practice
9(1):33–39

Williamson G, Dodds S 1999 The effectiveness
of a group approach to clinical supervision
in reducing stress: a review of the
literature. Journal of Clinical Nursing
8:338–344

Yegdich T 1999 Lost in the crucible of
supportive clinical supervision: supervision
is not therapy. Journal of Advanced
Nursing 29(5):1265–1275

4 THE CONTINUING CHALLENGE OF CLINICAL SUPERVISION

9

Some ideas and approaches in implementing clinical supervision in practice

John Driscoll

INTRODUCTION

Whether you are a clinician, manager, or organizational executive there comes a point at which the image of what clinical supervision might look like in clinical practice needs to move from a vague theory into some form of workable reality. Without doubt, as described in Chapter 1, the stakes have been raised by clinical governance which demands workable systems of staff support and continuing professional development (CPD), of which clinical supervision is now becoming a fundamental and legitimate part. This has implications for healthcare organizations, as it will mean periodically reviewing the infrastructure for what is already happening with clinical supervision, actively getting started at a departmental level, or seriously considering where to start when implementing clinical supervision across an organization.

This chapter begins at stimulating reflection on why a clinician has to change the way they work already and offers a pragmatic approach to getting clinical supervision off the ground at an individual and departmental level before considering the 'problems' of organizational implementation. A key to the sustainability of implementing clinical supervision is to involve healthcare professionals right from the start so that they can actively contribute to how it could work in areas of practice. Despite the organizational challenges posed by implementing clinical supervision in practice, I would suggest a wonderful opportunity now exists to open up multiprofessional conversations across the organization to really embed clinical supervision as part of everyday practice. Fortunately, rather than perhaps unfortunately, there is not one single method or format for the implementation of clinical supervision (Lucas et al 2000), because of the diverse and complex nature of healthcare delivery.

Based on my personal experiences in supporting the implementation of clinical supervision (often as an 'outsider' or external to healthcare organizations) I observe that frequently interdisciplinary rivalries, an unwillingness to share supervision experiences, resources and expertise and the continuance of multiple professional and organizational policies only seem to serve to disable, rather than enable, clinical supervision.

In this respect I agree with Cottrell's (2002) analysis that the organizational challenge of implementing clinical supervision is not that dissimilar to engaging in clinical supervision itself. In other words it needs to begin with acknowledging the importance of attending to the basic roles, responsibilities and expectations of those who will be affected by the initiative.

Is it too obvious to state that enabling collaboration within organizations helps them to withstand the inevitable challenges and sustain the initiative of implementation of any major change, but more specifically clinical supervision? Perhaps the implementation of clinical supervision in a healthcare organization, despite being on people's minds and impossible to ignore, could be likened to the metaphor of the 'elephant in the room'. In this situation, despite its obviousness, it fails to get 'noticed' perhaps because nobody knows quite what to do with the enormity of it or everybody hopes that it will simply go away!

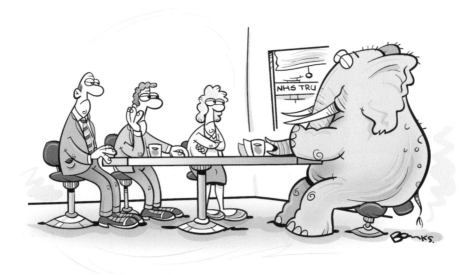

Acknowledging the elephant's presence in the organization is likely to be helpful in the first instance to challenge perceptions and potentially offer new opportunities to change the way work is currently undertaken. But why change the way you work already to include clinical supervision as part of your everyday activities?

WHY CHANGE THE WAY YOU WORK TO INCORPORATE CLINICAL SUPERVISION?

While accepting that clinical supervision may mean different things for different people and professions, the three main components of supervision in healthcare practice summarized in Chapter 1 were:

■ Supervised practice and learning.

■ Organizational supervision.

■ Supportive supervision.

Clinical supervision is considered to be the latter, being primarily a form of supportive supervision for qualified healthcare professionals, contributing to their learning and continued professional development and differentiated from more managerial forms of supervision. It has been likened to a formal and regular professional conversation (Launer 2003:94), but unlike some of those other supervisory processes, clinical supervision sets out not to be the kind of conversation that involves giving people advice, assessing them or solving their problems for them, but one in which space, time and professional support is provided to reflect on encounters with patients/clients or professional relationships.

A starting point in considering individually changing the way you work to incorporate clinical supervision might be to consider the questions contained in Box 9.1.

BOX 9.1	*Some individual questions to consider when contemplating the value of clinical supervision for your own practice*

■ Do you feel supported at work?

■ Do you have a regular opportunity to get some feedback or discuss practice concerns in confidence as a qualified health professional?

■ Does your organization have a policy on clinical supervision?

■ What are the organizational expectations for you and clinical supervision emerging from such a policy?

■ What does your professional organization say about the need for clinical supervision?

■ What are the professional expectations for you and clinical supervision?

■ What might be the impact for you, or your colleagues, if there is little organizational or professional support available to you in practice?

■ What might be the implications for continuing to be in a form of supervision (assuming you are already) that you consider ineffective?

Some of the questions posed ask you to consider whether clinical supervision is taking place with a view to you becoming involved or starting the process, and assume that for some, no mechanism is available or happens infrequently. Under clinical governance in the UK, while clinical supervision is promoted as a legitimate work-based support and development activity for qualified health professionals, this might not yet have been translated into a workable organizational policy. This will be less likely in the future, with many professional organizations in healthcare already aligning themselves to support CPD initiatives and developing (or have already developed) policies or guidelines as part of the periodic professional registration process (BAAT 2005, BDA 2000, COT 1997, CSP 2005, NMC 2002, NQ-ANZCMHN 2000, RCSLT 1996, ScoR 2003a, 2003b).

I am often asked why there is a need to have clinical supervision when there appear to be informal support networks more immediately available in practice for healthcare professionals. Some emerge almost intuitively, from working with and knowing that you can trust particular people who are prepared to listen to your concerns. Such informal peer support is often used as a way of letting colleagues share in stressful clinical experiences and a natural part of the working day, playing a vital part in coping with everyday professional practice. As was previously stated in Chapter 1, while not exactly clinical supervision, these informal and 'ad-hoc' meetings or support networks can reduce professional isolation but are often based on a 'chance meeting' or are immediate 'responses to' something that is happening or has happened. In the experience of O'Riordan (2002) and Cleary and Freeman (2005), implementing clinical supervision can be perceived as a threat to those informal networks at work contributing to a culture of passive resistance to getting started at all.

Based on what you have read and your understandings about clinical supervision:
- In what ways do you think that clinical supervision could be perceived as a threat to your own informal support networks in practice?
- How might this manifest itself in developing clinical supervision?
- What would need to happen to lessen the clinical supervision threat in practice to aid its development?

One wonders how possible it is to be able to *adapt* an informal support network as clinical supervision, rather than *adopt* other people's ideas about clinical supervision. As Smith (1995) rightly asserted over a decade ago:

> ... although clinical supervision may be needed in clinical practice it also has to be wanted by practitioners ...

My personal experience leads me to believe that it is possible to develop a clinical supervision relationship from what is an informal network. For me, it simply started with talking to somebody I trusted and respected on an ad-hoc basis and became more formalized, with an agreement made to meet regularly every four weeks. Although a concern might be that it is more difficult to challenge someone you like, the development of clinical supervision gave us the chance to review what we already did but 'raised the bar higher' so there was more substance, regularity and purpose to our conversations. It might be interesting if a possibility exists in your own practice to try to develop a clinical supervision relationship from an informal network. Prior to making such a commitment you might wish to visit the previous chapters by Stephen Power and Daniel Nicholls.

One has to also acknowledge that change is challenging within our personal, let alone professional, lives. For instance try:

- sleeping on the opposite side of the bed to your partner for two weeks,
- reading a book instead of watching the television in the evening,

(My own particular failure was ... flossing teeth after each meal following a visit to the dentist!)

In either of the above, it is important that you as an individual can perceive, or see some likely benefits for, the change. If you do, you are much more likely to commit that change. So it is with clinical supervision; healthcare professionals will not commit to a change in practice that does not seem to offer benefits and has obvious implications for the way clinical supervision is initially presented to health professionals. Often it will not be the clinical supervision itself that causes the resistance to change, but what might need to be different as a consequence of it being introduced. A very normal reaction to introducing something new (like sleeping on the wrong side of the bed) is to try and preserve the past, rather than being propelled out of our own comfort zones in practice and into uncertainty and challenge. Interestingly, as Wilkin and colleagues (1997) remind us:

> ... within the paradox that change is the only thing likely to remain constant in healthcare lies the irony that the object of resistance — clinical supervision, could actually provide some relief from the pressures such changes have created ...

I am beginning to become less surprised by the number of healthcare professionals who readily state opinions to others about the value (or not) of engaging in clinical supervision when they have never experienced it for themselves. For me it is only then that you can really have any firm ideas about what clinical supervision is like. While acknowledging that the ideal situation is for the organization to have a suitable infrastructure in place to get started with clinical supervision, for me, not having this need not stop healthcare professionals from simply experiencing it for themselves within the resources already available at their disposal.

GETTING STARTED BY EXPERIENCING CLINICAL SUPERVISION IN THE DEPARTMENT

This section moves from the individual confronted by the change and challenge of clinical supervision to suggesting some practical ideas for small groups of health professionals in a department to get going together in lieu of any organizational intentions on the horizon. Often I hear from different health professionals that their organization has not yet started to implement a system of clinical supervision, when clearly there is a willingness to do so. My own response is to encourage groups or individuals to just get started; providing that there is some sort of basic idea about what clinical supervision sets out to do, a general consensus can be reached and the departmental head is consulted. Another way of reframing clinical supervision within a department might be to consider it not just in terms of individual outcomes or benefits as health professionals, but as a process for contributing to improving the overall quality of healthcare delivery to patients or clients. The clinical governance mandate for healthcare organizations to have support and CPD mechanisms in place for health professionals would seem to permit those in practice to at least get started with clinical supervision, even if no formalized system is yet up and running.

A distinct advantage of working together to develop clinical supervision at grass roots in the department is that the resistance often caused by imposing change from top down and the subsequent lack of ownership is significantly reduced (Price & Chalker 2000).

Clinical supervision will necessarily involve the allocation of planned time and other resources during working hours for the activity, and this does *not* include the time needed to prepare for its implementation in the department beforehand!

Inevitably, this means that there will be cost and logistical implications in trying to cover busy workloads to facilitate clinical supervision happening. Therefore a meeting with the departmental head is an essential beginning. There are at least five good reasons for doing so (Box 9.2).

BOX 9.2	*Five reasons why you need to consult a departmental head before commencing clinical supervision*

- Your departmental head needs to endorse the activity, as it involves allocation of resources — it is no good staff feeling supported at work if there are no staff in the department to look after patients
- Departmental heads will have already heard about clinical supervision and, unknown to you, may already be helping with strategic plans for the initiative within the organization
- You can formally declare your own interest in clinical supervision and this may lead to formally networking with others in your organization who share a similar interest
- Departmental heads can support you in managing the implementation of clinical supervision as they are likely to have a wide experience of change management at local level
- Departmental heads will know through their own networks who you can liaise with in order to share learning and experiences, e.g. networking with a neighbouring organization to see how clinical supervision is operating already, or funding staff attendance at relevant study days

While there would seem no professional argument about setting up departmental or local systems of clinical supervision, translating this into the everyday practice is likely to be more challenging. Do not be surprised if your own enthusiasm for clinical supervision, stemming from an introductory workshop organized by your educational provider or professional organization or just reading around the subject, is not met with the same enthusiasm from colleagues who were working in the department in your absence and do not know as much about it as you.

The first stage of launching clinical supervision after meeting with the departmental head is to generate a critical awareness of clinical supervision and disseminate information about the possibilities and options that exist for the department. Stimulating a discussion about what clinical supervision is and is not will be enormously helpful in preparing the ground about how you and your colleagues intend going about it. It is very likely that there will already be varying levels of expertise to hand in the department. Organizing some regular meetings with colleagues to focus on a number of key issues prior to commencing clinical supervision in the department is likely to be necessary (Box 9.3).

BOX 9.3	*Key issues that will need to be raised with staff colleagues prior to commencing clinical supervision in your department*

- Gaining a shared departmental understanding about clinical supervision
- Gaining support from colleagues for introducing clinical supervision
- Agreeing on key roles such as lead person(s) who will assume responsibility
- The purpose of introducing clinical supervision to the department
- What resources will be required, including finding the time and attendance at training or awareness events
- Who the supervisors and supervisees will be and why
- What to include in any contract or agreement
- How to access clinical supervisors, e.g. internal or external
- What the likely format(s) will be, e.g. one-to-one, group
- Where it will take place
- Confidentiality and documentation
- What to do with those who do not wish to be involved in the initiative
- How it will be evaluated for its effectiveness
- Drawing up a departmental position statement based on any existing organizational policies on clinical supervision

Although you might think that this part of implementing clinical supervision is too time-consuming for the department, it is essential to be clear not only about the direction in which you intend to travel, but just as importantly, what form other people in the department think clinical supervision should take. This will save time when confronted by the inevitable challenges that occur that will test the resilience of the department later on in the implementation project. Having an external person to guide the preliminary meetings can be useful to ensure that the limited time is used effectively and to mediate any differences of opinion. Obviously, it is essential that all meetings are documented or recorded in some way, as they will be taking place during working hours. Capturing what is going on not only serves as an *aide-mémoire*, but provides on going evidence of the process, and the lessons being learned and help to maintain direction. Implementing clinical supervision within a department can be likened to some of the exploits of those pioneering balloonists who tried to be the first to circumnavigate the globe (Figure 9.1).

I am sure that all the competitors wanted to be the first to get from point A to point B but their chances of getting there directly were remote, given the variable air currents, wind speeds, climate and available technologies. In reality, the intended direction of the balloonist was unlikely to be the actual route taken. What the balloonist requires is courage, skill and enough flexibility to foresee the dangers and variables that exist, while at the same time not losing sight of the ultimate objective, point B!

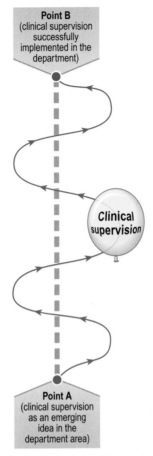

Figure 9.1　A likely route for implementing clinical supervision in the department

Using the balloon analogy, you might wish to reflect on how you and your colleagues in the department have already managed change previously, e.g. meeting performance targets, incorporating care pathways, incorporating evidence-based practice. For instance, how did you get from point A to point B? What sorts of things temporarily blew you off the main course that you were heading towards? How did you manoeuvre back on course again? So it is with clinical supervision; you cannot embark on the journey without adequate back-up and support and some idea of the variables that you are likely to face along the way and what to do when you get blown off course. Like that of the balloonist, the journey may be a bit turbulent, and making the wrong decisions can bring you back to earth with a bump, as well as having some professional bruises to show for having engaged in the venture! Prior to launch it can be useful to think of the 'forces' necessary to get the clinical supervision project balloon airborne in your department as well as maintain its direction.

Leigh (2001:174) describes the 'forces' at play that challenge the *status quo* of a department with implementing change such as clinical supervision. The forces that will continually counteract each other are described as *driving forces* (those that will get and keep you airborne along your intended clinical supervision route) and *restraining forces* (those that will blow you off your intended clinical supervision route).

- Photocopy Figure 9.2 and sit down with your colleagues to begin to notice the different forces that are likely to interact with each other when you are implementing clinical supervision in your department.
- Together as a group discuss some change that has happened in your own department recently and how the different forces were managed.
- Based on this discussion, compile a list of some the forces likely to be present in each of the quadrants when implementing clinical supervision.

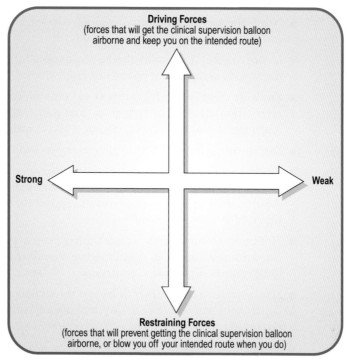

Figure 9.2 Noticing the forces that exist when considering implementing clinical supervision in your department

Having considered some of the driving and restraining forces in your practice area, to begin the process and then continue in the right direction, three things are likely to need to happen, which will form a structure for your ongoing discussions and departmental implementation plan:

- The driving forces for clinical supervision, once identified, need to be strengthened.

- The restraining forces for clinical supervision, once identified, need to be weakened.

- You might also wish to consider some additional driving forces to the ones you have already identified.

Obviously if the driving forces are stronger than the restraining forces your clinical supervision balloon will be likely not only to become airborne but to remain

moving in the right direction. If not, then the clinical supervision implementation plan will urgently need reviewing. It is much better to build regular reviews
into the implementation process to avoid this sense of 'crisis', which in itself
might be considered a restraining force.

You may wish to compare, or get some ideas of, some of the likely driving
and restraining forces for implementing clinical supervision in the department in
Figure 9.3.

You can probably think of some additional driving forces that will keep the
department close to its intended direction of implementing clinical supervision.
For instance:

■ Not being too overambitious; you have to learn to fly the balloon before you
  can attempt to circumnavigate the world!

■ Identifying key staff willing to be responsible for carrying out one or more of
  the actions arising from your team discussions.

■ Ensuring there is an adequate way to communicate with all staff, e.g. those
  on rotation, days off or annual leave or part-timers, so they can have
  information about what is going on with clinical supervision.

■ Documenting the progress of clinical supervision in the department.

■ Working closely with the departmental manager to ensure 'quick wins', e.g.
  targeting those in the department who are committed to the process, setting
  departmental appraisal objectives to support the implementation of clinical
  supervision throughout the year

■ Not being afraid to network with other people with more experience in
  clinical supervision, e.g. neighbouring organizations or departments such as
  local education providers, professional bodies, authors of journal articles.

■ Setting feasible timeframes to launch the clinical supervision balloon in the
  department and where necessary making adjustments to emerging
  restraining forces that blow you off course.

Inevitably, as with any intended change in practice, there will be resistance. Broadly
speaking, resistance is a way of saying 'No!' to change. But when handled sensitively, because you had planned and prepared for it, resistance can make a valuable contribution to the successful implementation of clinical supervision. In
order to weaken any forces resisting your implementation of clinical supervision, it is better to understand why they are occurring, rather than react in a
hostile or defensive way to them.

In my opinion, it can sometimes be useful for the team to be honest enough
to say at the outset to the departmental manager 'at this point, with our existing
resources, we are not able to give our best attention to getting clinical supervision started'. This will prevent you from setting off in a piecemeal way only to
see the initiative fall flat on its face. However, one of the exciting things about
just getting started with clinical supervision is that initially it will be experimental and the ways that it is carried out will vary. For instance, it might be
more cost-effective to consider working as a group in clinical supervision and is
discussed in more detail in another chapter.

Although clinical supervision 'training' is an important element to consider
in the organizational implementation of clinical supervision and discussed in the
next section, I think it is perfectly possible not to have to have a deep theoretical

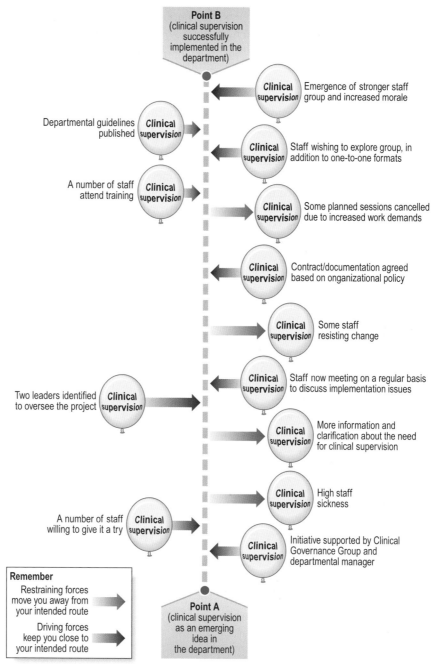

Figure 9.3 Some likely driving and restraining forces for implementing clinical supervision in your department

knowledge at the outset for what is essentially having a formalized professional conversation with a colleague about the situation you find yourself in at work. If clinical supervision is viewed from the start as a learning situation not only about your clinical work but also about implementing it throughout the department, challenges can then become learning opportunities rather than a chance to criticize.

No two departments will implement clinical supervision in the same way, as needs change and healthcare arenas can be very different. What is important is to document and openly discuss and act upon the lessons being learned with a view to then developing further clinical supervision skills at a point forward.

In my view, it is a myth to think that without any formal 'training', clinical supervision cannot begin in some rudimentary or temporary way in a department, provided there is a commitment to experimenting with it, and one or two individuals already have a working knowledge of the process. The development of clinical supervision skills is a lifelong journey that cannot be adequately fulfilled by attending a short training programme or studying a module or two at a university. For instance, supervisory skills learned also need to be sustained and refined in practice. Again, from personal experience, only practising regular clinical supervision, particularly as a supervisor, begins to reveal the full extent and potential for clinical supervision in practice.

Up to this point, this section has focused on simply 'getting started' with local clinical supervision schemes which demand minimal organizational resources, but in an ideal world there would be a commitment to the development and implementation of clinical supervision across the whole organization *before* there was an attempt to get it started in any particular department.

You now might have a better working knowledge of getting going in your own department, but remember that to launch and sustain a clinical supervision balloon across your whole organization could be much more complicated. However, many of the principles remain the same whether implementing in an organization or in a department. It is perhaps obvious that the stakes are higher when investing in an initiative across an organization, where to get it wrong would be very wasteful in terms of resources, but what can be even more counterproductive is the effect of failure on staff; they can often be left with an intensely negative attitude towards the very concept of clinical supervision, jeopardizing the potential practice improvements in patient and client care it could have brought about.

LARGE-SCALE IMPLEMENTATION OF CLINICAL SUPERVISION ACROSS THE HEALTHCARE ORGANIZATION

Having been privileged to have been personally involved in supporting many clinical supervision implementation schemes over the last decade, an immediate metaphor that comes to mind is the consumption of either 'instant' or 'percolated' coffee. Some organizations obviously governed by limited resources, lack of understanding, the annual clinical governance report or the pressure to tick a performance indicator box might prefer the 'instant' coffee solution. Without a thought for how it is served, it is gulped down regardless of taste, before moving on to the next round of must do's. Under these circumstances the implications of implementing clinical supervision will not have been thoroughly thought through; it is simply instituted as a 'quick fix', a 'means to an end', and is rarely sustainable in the long term, as aptly described by Robinson (2005):

> ... the Trust did not offer a training programme for clinical supervisors, so experienced staff who had acted as mentors and preceptors were asked to

volunteer as supervisors with the intention that the training be arranged at a later date ...

In contrast, the making and taking of percolated coffee cannot be rushed, often requires a suitable environment and can be part of a special occasion that is conducive to talking and listening. Not unlike the extensive range of coffees available to suit wide-ranging palates, there are a range of approaches in implementing clinical supervision:

- training needs analysis (Gallinagh 2000),
- goals and objectives (McKeown & Thompson 2001),
- action learning (Freshwater et al 2003, RCNI 2000, WMCSLS 1998),
- action research (Lyon 1999),
- problem-solving (Rogers & Topping Morris 1997, Wright 1989:7), or
- force field analyses (Leigh 2001:174).

Any one of these approaches could have been utilized to manage the project described above by Robinson (2005).

In the process of implementing clinical supervision there are rich seams of inevitable barriers or problems to consider when devising a workable strategy across an organization. You might wish to compare those in Box 9.4 with some of your own initial ideas about the setting of priorities in getting started.

BOX 9.4   *Some likely barriers or problems to consider with large-scale implementation of clinical supervision*

- Negative attitudes by enough staff to have an impact on widespread implementation (Cleary & Freeman 2005, Dixon & Bramwell 2001, Hughes & Morcom 1998)
- Lack of understanding about clinical supervision by staff (Smith 2001) and managers (Ask & Roche 2005)
- Concerns about maintaining confidentiality (Clough 2003)
- Supervisee perceptions of clinical supervision being a system of management control (Burrows 1995, Ask & Roche 2005)
- Cost implications (Pateman 1998:187, Bishop 1998:14, Nolan & Smit 2001:181)
- Resource implications, e.g. finding extra time and a suitable environment in clinical practice (CSP 2005, Duarri & Kendrick 1999, Lucas et al 2000, McKeown & Thompson 2001, Teasdale 2000, White & Winstanley 2003)
- Defining the term 'supervision' (Bush 2005, Clough 2003, Wright et al 1997)
- Lack of trained supervisors (Lucas et al 2000, Robinson 2005, Smith 2001), feelings of inadequacy as a new supervisor (Rafferty & Coleman 2001), difficulties in maintaining a pool of supervisors (Price & Chalker 2000)

Although some of the common barriers to the organizational implementation of clinical supervision have been identified, the literature is only just beginning to recognize how the organization itself can contribute to compromising, instead of actively co-operating with, the development of clinical supervision. For instance, Grant (2003) asserts that often organizations have an implicit rule that innovations, such as clinical supervision, should not upset existing structures or custom and practice. This has often meant organizations adopting an 'instant coffee' solution through implementing 'in-house' schemes (cascading the delivery of clinical supervision through managerial lines of command), directly contradicting the spirit of the concept of implementation in which health professionals are expected to shape its meaning, uptake and delivery with managerial *support*, rather than, as Weaver (2001) states, management *control* or *interference*.

Cottrell (2002) in one of the first detailed publications challenging how an organization can limit the development of clinical supervision warned:

> ... despite the potential of clinical supervision to open up traditionally closed systems of practice to compassionate critique, and so to intervene meaningfully and directly upon the process of care delivery, many attempts to introduce clinical supervision seem to either fall at the first hurdle, end in crisis of one form or another, or tend to slowly 'peter out' over time.

He describes how an organization can unconsciously (or consciously) sabotage the implementation of clinical supervision through collusive supervisory relationships that can occur within the organization (Figure 9.4), resulting in:

- 'Token supervision' (when the organization and the manager collude).
- 'Local resistance' (when the supervisee and the manager collude).
- 'Mutinous supervision' (when the supervisees and supervisors collude).
- 'Suspicion position' (when the organization and supervisors collude).

a) Read Cottrell S 2002 Suspicion, resistance, tokenism and mutiny: problematic dynamics relevant to the implementation of clinical supervision in nursing. Journal of Psychiatric and Mental Health Nursing 9:667–671. Alternatively you can access online at http://www.clinical-supervision.com/article.htm

b) Do you agree with how an organization might collude to limit the development of clinical supervision? How do you think the article might resonate with your own organizational attempts at setting up clinical supervision and what might be the implications?

c) Make brief notes on how, in your opinion, your organization might need to move from:
   - 'Tokenism' to Commitment for clinical supervision
   - 'Resistance' to Acceptance of clinical supervision
   - 'Mutiny' to Loyalty with clinical supervision
   - 'Suspicion' to Trust with clinical supervision

Some obvious ways of reducing organizational problems are to be transparent with the development of clinical supervision and to move away from a traditional hierarchical implementation approach, sometimes referred to as 'top down', to one that is more 'bottom up' and inclusive of practitioners. While differing approaches have their merits, the development of clinical supervision will naturally involve managers who need to be actively resourcing and supporting the process, with practitioners developing the process within their own departmental realities. Another way of maintaining transparency in the implementation of clinical supervision is to develop a collaborative or multiprofessional approach to its implementation from the start (Ask & Roche 2005, CSP 2005, Townend

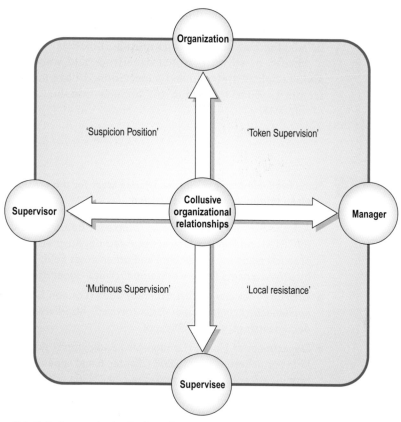

Figure 9.4 Collusive organizational relationships

2005) in step with current healthcare reforms taking place. The key to successfully collaborating is in giving a voice to all those who will be likely to be affected by its implementation and establishing an open and ongoing dialogue. For example, the facilitation of well thought out and representative 'Awareness Workshops' for a cross-section of the workforce *before* the process begins not only serves to identify potential issues and concerns (Box 9.4), but also provides an opportunity to share experiences and help to make clinical supervision more sustainable in the longer term. Spence et al (2002) suggest that the initial content of collaborative 'Awareness Workshops' might need to:

- Explore the concept of clinical supervision.
- Examine its advantages and disadvantages for implementing in practice.
- Discuss the various approaches and formats that might be used.
- Explore some of the key issues that the organization will face with implementation.

You can probably think of other things to include, such as devising an organizational briefing paper for participants, bringing in those who already have some expertise from a neighbouring organization or profession or discussing your needs with your local education provider. A number of healthcare organizations have also published online clinical supervision implementation guidelines that suggest where to start and include pathways to further illustrate possibilities that might be adapted for your own organization (Box 9.5).

Finally, based on personal experience and some of the literature available about implementing clinical supervision, I have summarized some of the key factors to consider within an organization for supporting its development (Table 9.1).

BOX 9.5	*Some available online resources offering ideas for the organizational implementation of clinical supervision*

- Ask and Roche (2005) National Centre for Education and Training on Addiction (NCETA) and Flinders University, Adelaide, Australia. Clinical supervision: a practical guide for the alcohol and other drugs field: http://www.nceta.flinders.edu.au/pdf/clinical-supervision/theguide.pdf
- Chartered Society of Physiotherapy 2005 (London, UK) (CPD 37) A guide to implementing clinical supervision (revised). http://www.csp.org.uk/uploads/documents/csp_cpd37_2005.pdf
- Department of Health (London, UK) Radiography skills mix: a report on the four tier delivery system 2003 Chapter 6 and appendix 6: clinical supervision http://www.eradiography.net/regsetc/Skill%20mix%20report.pdf#search='strategies%20for%20implementing%20clinical%20supervision'
- Department of Health (Leeds, UK) Making a difference: clinical supervision in primary care 2000 http://www.dh.gov.uk/assetroot/04/06/15/20/04061520.pdf
- Freshwater D, Storey L, Walsh L 2003 Establishing clinical supervision in prison healthcare settings (Foundation of Nursing Studies, London, UK) http://www.fons.org/ns/Dissemination_series_reports/Diss%20Series%20Vol%201%20No%207.pdf
- McKinley and Pegram 1999 Implementing a model of clinical supervision (Foundation of Nursing Studies, London, UK) http://www.fons.org/ahcp/archive/pdfs/Implementing%20CS.pdf
- Nursing and Midwifery Advisory Group 2004 Clinical supervision guidelines for mental health nurses in Northern Ireland: best practice guidelines (Department of Health, Social Services and Public Safety, Belfast, UK) http://www.dhsspsni.gov.uk/clinical_supervision.pdf

General ideas about clinical supervision:

http://www.clinical-supervision.com

http://www.online-supervision.net

http://www.supervisionandcoaching.com

(Other information about the organizational implementation of clinical supervision can be found in Barriball et al 2004, Bassett 1999, Bond & Holland 1998, Cutcliffe et al 2001, Hussain 2004, Kohner 1994, RCNI 2000, SCoR 2003a, Spence 2002, WMCSLS 1998.)

TABLE 9.1 *A summary of key factors to consider in developing an organizational clinical supervision strategy*

	Key factor(s) for developing an organizational strategy for clinical supervision	Examples/actions
S	Support roles identified	– Clinical supervision facilitators/leads/ champions – Senior management team/project steering group
U	Use of an evaluative framework for project and monitoring effectiveness of clinical supervision afterwards	– Build in periodic reviews with appropriate feedback loops within organization – Use of education provider(s) – Research & Development/audit input
P	Purposely being aware of political and professional agendas for implementation prior to commencement	– Consider appropriate change management strategy from expertise already in the organization – External networking/professional bodies
E	Education for increased understanding about clinical supervision	– Awareness raising workshops – Supervisor and supervisee development – Liaise with local education or external providers
R	Resources bid for and secured prior to commencement of project	– Executive, management, clinical and administrative – Secure adequate funding for pilot project and beyond
V	'Vision-ing' clinical supervision with stakeholders and throughout organization	– Develop a shared vision of clinical supervision, e.g. workshops/focus groups/ action learning sets/interviews
I	Identification of any previous clinical supervision policy, guidelines and documentation in the organization or professional bodies	– Acknowledge previous attempts made – Map what is already happening and effectiveness – Emphasize confidentiality and how this will be maintained
S	Support for practising supervisors and those actively engaged in support roles	– Formation of clinical supervision steering group – Group supervision for supervisors – Action learning approach
I	Incentives for finding the time to engage in the clinical supervision process	– Active managerial support for clinical supervision time – Celebrate and promote success – Support for training – Recognize effort
O	Ownership through organizational openness	– Devolve but support responsible autonomy in practice

TABLE 9.1 *(cont'd)*

Key factor(s) for developing an organizational strategy for clinical supervision		Examples/actions
		– Build in a consultation process prior to commencing – Allow practitioners to devise their own solutions e.g. experiment with different formats – Facilitate departmental adaptation of organizational policy and guidelines
N	Neutralizing staff suspicions and concerns	– Acknowledge concerns at the outset – Differentiate between clinical and managerial forms of supervision – Clarify organizational expectations – Develop enough working supervisors to allow choice – Promote a collaborative and inter-professional approach

Other priority areas to consider:

AN 'APPRECIATIVE' APPROACH TO THE 'PROBLEMS' OF IMPLEMENTING CLINICAL SUPERVISION

You might be forgiven at this stage of the chapter for not only having a sense of being overwhelmed by the prospect of implementing clinical supervision with all its inherent problems and difficulties but also of having a lurking suspicion that this book is suggesting that there is a 'proper' way of doing clinical supervision based on ideas and theories of people external to the organization — and that I could be one of those people, providing yet more ideas, unappreciative of the practicalities of implementing clinical supervision in everyday clinical practice! Not so.

Of course if we simply focus on the gloomy nature of implementing clinical supervision, which is often based on what is *not* happening, it inevitably generates further gloom and fosters a sense of helplessness, and not surprisingly, like a self-fulfilling prophecy, things go wrong.

In1999, at a Reflective Practice Symposium at the Royal Society of Medicine in London, I participated in the discussions on 'Appreciative Inquiry', an alternative method to the traditional problem-solving approach. (Here I need to acknowledge Barbara Gaskell and Ann Girling, who I have worked with since on a number of initiatives in facilitating 'modified' appreciative approaches supporting the implementation of clinical supervision in organizations.) What I have learned, and continue to learn, about facilitating an appreciative approach is that if I intentionally seek out positive feelings, promote learning and celebrate success in groups or with individuals, very often they find value in what they are doing. Perhaps it is stating the obvious, but people are more willing to engage and be open about success and positive things. Therefore adopting an 'appreciative approach' provides the clinical supervision implementer not only with an approach to change, but an opportunity to reframe people's stance with regard to that change. By this, I mean that by being deliberately hopeful, working with optimism and breaking free from the endless cycles of problems leading to even more problems that just seem to demoralize and continually sap the energy of practitioners, the appreciative approach constructively motivates practitioners.

My intention here is not to get bogged down with the theory of appreciative inquiry but to concentrate on its application to the implemention of clinical supervision. But first two questions posed by Sue Annis-Hammond (1998:6):

- What problems are you having?
- What is working around here?

She asserts that those two questions underline the difference between traditional change management theory and appreciative inquiry. A traditional change approach to implementing clinical supervision looks for the problem(s) (many of which have already been identified in this chapter), diagnoses what is happening and then treats the problem(s). Not a surprising approach to be adopted by healthcare professionals who day in day out problem solve, diagnose and treat. However, if we move away from patient care and apply this approach to making changes in practice, for example, implementing clinical supervision, we end up looking for problems and inevitably find them (Box 9.4).

David Cooperrider and his associates at Case Western University in Ohio challenged this approach in the mid-seventies and introduced the concept of appreciative inquiry (Cooperrider & Whitney 1999, Cooperrider et al 2003, Watkins & Mohr 2001). As the term suggests, to 'appreciate' is to increase in value, and with appreciative inquiry (AI) the emphasis is on looking for what works in an organization and describing 'where the organization wants to be' based on describing 'special moments' of where they have been. Because the statements are grounded in real experiences and history, people know how to repeat their successes. A comparison of the two approaches, in relation to implementing clinical supervision, is offered in Table 9.2; there is a suggestion of choice between using a 'problem-focused' approach or 'possibility-focused' approach to implementation.

TABLE 9.2 *Fundamental differences between a problem-solving and an appreciative approach to implementing clinical supervision in the organization*

Problem-solving approach to implementing clinical supervision	Appreciative approach to implementing clinical supervision
A 'felt' need to identify 'problems'	Appreciating and valuing the best of 'what is already happening'
Analysing the cause of those 'problems'	Envisioning 'what might be'
Action planning to 'treat' the 'problems'	Discussing 'what should be'
Basic assumption:	**Basic assumption:**
Clinical supervision as 'problems' to be resolved to achieve implementation	Clinical supervision as a mystery to be embraced to achieve implementation

Rossi (2006), in an overview of AI comparing the two approaches, asserted that AI does not ignore problems but recognizes them as a desire for something else. An AI approach then works to identify and enhance that 'something else'. In clinical supervision workshops, using this approach, I will acknowledge that there are perceived problems in implementing clinical supervision and 'park' them on a flipchart for reframing at a later stage.

Of course there are times when it is not helpful to even suggest an AI approach, for example, in healthcare organizations that favour more hierarchical or 'top down' approaches. In such organizations there is little desire and no time allocated for dreaming and designing a clinical supervision scheme in a collaborative way.

Other organizations might see this approach as threatening once the 'penny has dropped' that it will require more resources (not only to initiate but also to sustain the clinical supervision schemes) and that clinical supervision, if it is to work, will be under the direct influence of the practitioners/participants themselves.

A number of models for AI have been developed since its inception and are available online. These, along with other excellent resources, are given in Box 9.6.

BOX 9.6	Selected AI resources available online
	http://appreciativeinquiry.case.edu/
	http://www.appreciative-inquiry.org/
	http://www.aradford.co.uk
	http://www.mellish.com.au/Resources/lizarticle.htm
	http://www.nickheap.co.uk/articles_by_cat.asp?ART_CAT_ID=27
	http://www.taosinstitute.net/appreciative/appreciative.html

A worked example of how a modified AI approach assisted the implementation of clinical supervision in North East London Mental Health Trust (NELMHT) was in the devising of a full-day AI workshop held at an external venue for around 50 multiprofessional participants in collaboration with senior management. The aim of the event was to work with participants to design an organizational clinical supervision strategy. The intentions of the AI workshop were:

- To obtain staff support for implementing clinical supervision in NELMHT using AI as a process for positive change.

- To discover and share what NELMHT could learn by inquiring into previous and current positive experiences and understandings about 'supervision'.

- To begin to capture 'best practice supervision' from a range of professional perspectives and discover how this can form the basis for the development of clinical supervision within NELMHT.

- To agree (in principle) a strategic 'way forward' that will include 'what needs to happen next' to ensure the continued development of clinical supervision within NELMHT.

The programme for the day (Figure 9.5) was structured around the 4 'D' Model (Watkins & Mohr 2001:43), which incorporated four phases: *Discovery/Dream/Design/Delivery*.

To begin with, participants interviewed each other in pairs and were asked to describe *one* really 'special supervisory moment' that had happened recently; one that participants felt had been supportive and resulted in a significant difference to what they had been trying to achieve in their practice. (At this stage, clinical supervision had not been introduced, although some were engaged in the process and had included it in their descriptions.) From each interview, two core factors were captured that in the participants' opinion had made that 'supervisory moment special'. Groups were then formed to compare and contrast their responses and identify what for them had made those supervisory moments special. Following a debriefing stage the core factors were described to the audience and listed on flipcharts as the 'best of what already is'. These lists were compared to the principles of clinical supervision as understood by the participants to give them an appreciation that some form of supervision already existed within NELMHT.

The afternoon was devoted to a creative exercise that celebrated what was already happening with 'supervision' and incorporated a number of affirmative statements based on the 'special moments': these were fed back to the senior management team to form the basis of a clinical supervision strategy. For example:

- We want NELMHT to create consistency in the undertaking of supervision across the Trust, while recognizing there will have to be differences.
- Every team in NELMHT should have an annual team away-day which is paid for and facilitated (adequate cover for the team being provided) because it is not just about individual development, it's about teams.
- Supervision is a continuous way of learning to enhance higher productivity, efficiency and morale.
- Clinical supervision should be available as a core component built into the job description of employees of NELMHT.
- NELMHT should develop a supervision policy that incorporates the importance of different styles of supervision that enhance the effectiveness of the team culture.

While more work by the facilitators might have produced more provocative statements, from a one day workshop enough energy was generated to produce not only the building blocks of a strategy, but also a number of volunteers who would then become the 'champions' of clinical supervision in the organization.

As a fundamental function of the AI approach is to continue to maintain the momentum and naturally raised expectations to support the actual delivery of the process, discussion sessions cannot be just 'talking shops' but have to be forums for action. In NELMHT the forum for action took the form of an externally facilitated working group that worked in depth on devising a suitable infrastructure and the publication of guidelines for clinical supervision that were largely based on the ideas from the original AI workshop (NELMHT 2005).

It would seem that an AI approach offers the possibility of an alternative to traditional methods of implementing clinical supervision. AI insists on identifying and then doing more of what is working well, rather than focusing on deficits and doing less of something that has presented a problem.

However, the AI approach will not suit all organizations, as it requires the willingness of the change agents and workshop participants to search for new possibilities to stretch the organizational potential and challenge traditional

North East London **NHS**

Mental Health NHS Trust

Developing a Strategy for Clinical Supervision through Noticing and Appreciating Supervisory Practice in NELMHT

0900–0915	**Coffee/registration and networking**
0915–0930	Welcome and Intentions for the day/Setting the scene for the development of clinical supervision in NELMHT
0930–0945	Appreciative Inquiry: clarifying this from more traditional change processes and setting the scene for the morning's activities
0945–1100	Appreciating past and present supervisory practice to inform clinical supervision in the organization (Paired and Group Exercises)
1100–1120	**Coffee and networking**
1120–1135	Debrief of the interview process
1135–1245	Capturing and Identifying 'best supervision practice in NELMHT' themes
1245–1300	Is clinical supervision happening already in NELMHT?
1300–1345	**Lunch and networking**
1345–1500	From Image to Action: using past and present practice to ensure best clinical supervision practice – A Declaration of Intentions for NELMHT (Exercise)
1500–1515	**Tea and networking**
1515–1545	Feedback/Group Declarations including action points for future workshops
1545–1600	Closing remarks...Closure and Evaluation

Figure 9.5 An AI-based workshop structure to develop an organizational strategy for clinical supervision

organizational hierarchies in implementing clinical supervision. The sense of ownership that emerges, based on personal narratives about what can and is already happening and then building on those foundations, for various reasons, may not be perceived as achievable by some.

There must be hundreds of different clinical supervision implementation stories in organizations just waiting to be told and all slightly different, there being no 'one fit all' format. The implications of adopting an AI approach are enormous for any organization; in relation to not just clinical supervision but any change initiative that requires a sense of ownership for its sustainability.

CONCLUSION

My intention with this chapter was to offer hope to those faced with the task of implementing clinical supervision in practice, as well as to outline a number of differing yet pragmatic approaches that can be used at different levels and that might be applicable within your organization. Perhaps the chapter might also help to liberate individuals from the conceptual chains of thinking that there is necessarily a 'right and proper way' to go about implementing clinical supervision. But I have pointed out that there are fundamental principles of execution for successful implementation and the key one of these is the adoption of a collaborative style involving honest and constructive conversations with each other.

You might wish to reflect on how the promotion of a more collaborative and multiprofessional approach to change initiatives in healthcare organizations is becoming the norm. Perhaps there has been so much change in professional healthcare that such approaches are simply taken for granted now and are not really noticed that much at all. I cannot help thinking that the development of clinical governance as a change initiative in its own right just a few years ago is a working example of individuals and departments surviving a systemic change in the way that healthcare organizations function and now beginning to flourish and innovate. I wonder whether all that previous learning, experience and subsequent development of expertise will now be brought to bear on actively supporting innovative clinical supervision schemes in those same healthcare organizations, while enabling practitioners to get on with the process themselves.

On reflection ... chapter summary

- Clinical supervision presents an organizational opportunity to establish multiprofessional conversations about its implementation.
- There is no one single method or format for implementing clinical supervision due to the complex nature of healthcare organizations.
- Healthcare professionals are unlikely to commit to a change like clinical supervision unless it is perceived to benefit their practice.
- Opportunities to collaborate with clinical supervision will promote a sense of ownership of the initiative and significantly reduce resistance.
- Acknowledging resistance to clinical supervision can make a valuable contribution to its implementation and stimulate further discussions on ways forward.
- An alternative approach to implementing clinical supervision is not to be overwhelmed by the 'problems' but focus on what already works as supervision and develop these ideas further.
- Developing an 'appreciative' approach to the implementation of clinical supervision promotes ownership as it is based on real narratives from clinical practice.

REFERENCES

Annis-Hammond S 1998 The thin book of appreciative inquiry. Thin Book, Plano, TX, USA

Ask A, Roche A 2005 Clinical supervision: a practical guide for the alcohol and other drugs field. National Centre for Education and Training on Addiction (NCETA) and Flinders University, Adelaide, Australia

BAAT 2005 Code of Ethics and Principles of Professional Practice for Arts Therapists. Online. Available at: http://www.baat.org/codeofethics.pdf#search='HPC%20supervision'. Accessed 10/2/06

Barriball L, While A, Munch U 2004 An audit of clinical supervision in primary care. British Journal of Community Nursing 9(9):389–397

Bassett C (ed) 1999 Clinical supervision: a guide for implementation. Nursing Times Books, London

BDA 2000 Guidance document clinical supervision for dieticians. British Dietetic Association (Dieticians). Online. Available at: http://members.bda.uk.com/Downloads/clinsuperdiet.pdf. Accessed 12/10/05

Bishop V 1998 Clinical supervision: what is it? In: Bishop V (ed) Clinical supervision in practice – some questions, answers and guidelines. Macmillan/Nursing Times Research, London, UK

Bond M, Holland S 1998 Skills of clinical supervision for nurses. Open University, Milton Keynes, UK

Burrows S 1995 Supervision: clinical development or management control? British Journal of Nursing 4(15):879–882

Bush T 2005 Overcoming the barriers to effective clinical supervision. Nursing Times 101(2):38–41

Cleary M, Freeman A 2005 The cultural realities of clinical supervision in an acute inpatient mental health setting. Issues in Mental Health Nursing 26:489–505

Clough A 2003 Clinical supervision in primary care. Primary Healthcare 13(9):15–18

COT 1997 Statement on supervision in occupational therapy SPP 150(A). College of Occupational Therapists, London

Cottrell S 2002 Suspicion, resistance, tokenism and mutiny: problematic dynamics relevant to the implementation of clinical supervision in nursing. Journal of Psychiatric and Mental Health Nursing 9:667–671

Cooperrider D, Whitney D 1999 Appreciative inquiry. Berrett-Koehler, San Francisco, CA, USA

Cooperrider D, Whitney D, Stavros J 2003 Appreciative inquiry handbook: the first in a series of AI workbooks for leaders of change. Lakeshore Communications & Berrett-Koehler, Bedford Heights, OH, USA

CSP 2005 A guide to implementing clinical supervision (information paper: CPD 37-revised). Chartered Society of Physiotherapy, London

Cutcliffe J, Butterworth T, Proctor B (eds) 2001 Fundamental themes in clinical supervision. Routledge, London

Dixon A, Bramwell R 2001 Neonatal nurses' attitudes to clinical supervision: results of a survey. Journal of Neonatal Nursing 7(1):20–24

DOH 2000 Making a difference: clinical supervision in primary care. Department of Health, London

Duarri W, Kendrick K 1999 Implementing clinical supervision. Professional Nurse 14(12):849–852

Freshwater D, Storey L, Walsh L 2003 Establishing clinical supervision in prison healthcare settings dissemination series (1) Foundation of Nursing Studies, London, UK

Gallinagh R 2000 Clinical supervision at work. Elderly Care 12(3):15–17

Grant A 2003 Opinion (clinical supervision). Mental Health Practice 6(6):22–23

Grant A 2000 Clinical supervision and organizational power: a qualitative study. Mental Health & Learning Disabilities 3(12):398–401

Hughes R, Morcom C 1998 Clinical supervision in a mental health in-patient area. Nursing Times Research 3(3):226–235

Hussain M 2004 Clinical supervision: implementing the framework from the College of Radiographers. Synergy (November):19–23

Kohner N 1994 Clinical supervision in practice. King's Fund Centre, London, UK

Launer J 2003 A narrative based approach to primary care supervision. In: Burton J, Launer J (eds) Supervision and support in primary care. Radcliffe Medical, Oxford, UK, p 91–101

Leigh A 2001 Force field analysis. In: Leigh A (ed) 20 ways to manage better. 3rd edn. Chartered Institute of Personnel and Development, London, UK

Lucas S, Jones A, Glover D 2000 Implementation problems. Nursing Times 96(11):49–52

Lyon J 1999 Applying Hart & Bond's typology: implementing clinical supervision in an acute setting. Nurse Researcher 6(2):39–56

McKeown C, Thompson J 2001 Implementing clinical supervision. Nursing Management 8(6):10–13

NELMHT 2005 Guidelines for clinical supervision. North East London Mental Health Trust, Ilford, London, UK

NMC 2002 Supporting nurses and midwives through lifelong learning. Nursing and Midwifery Council, London

Nolan M, Smit S 2001 Maintaining quality care in the independent sector. In: Cutcliffe J, Butterworth T, Proctor B (eds) Fundamental themes in clinical supervision. Routledge, London, UK, p 170–184

NQ-ANZCMHN 2000 Clinical supervision in psychiatric mental health nursing. North Queensland sub-branch of the Australia and New Zealand College of Mental Health Nurses. position statement on Supervision. Online. Available at: http://www.nq-anzcmhn.org. Accessed 11/1/06

Open University 1998 Clinical supervision: a development pack for nurses (K509). Open University, Buckingham, UK

O'Riordan B 2002 Why nurses choose not to undertake clinical supervision – the findings from one ICU. Nursing in Critical Care 7(2):59–66

Pateman B 1998 Clinical supervision in district nursing. In: Butterworth T, Faugier J, Burnard P (eds) Clinical supervision and mentorship in nursing. 2nd edn. Stanley Thornes, Cheltenham, UK, p 174–188

Price AM, Chalker M 2000 Our journey with clinical supervision in an intensive care unit. Intensive and Critical Care Nursing 16:51–55

Rafferty M, Coleman M 2001 Developmental transitions towards effective educational preparation for clinical supervision. In: Cutcliffe J, Butterworth T, Proctor B (eds) Fundamental themes in clinical supervision. Routledge, London, UK, p 84–95

RCNI 2000 Realising clinical effectiveness and clinical governance through clinical supervision (open learning pack). Royal College of Nursing Institute, Radcliffe Medical, Abingdon, Oxon, UK

RCSLT 1996 Communicating quality 2 – professional standards for speech and language therapists. Royal College of Speech and Language Therapists, London, UK

Robinson J 2005 Improving practice through a system of clinical supervision. Nursing Times 101(23):30–32

Rogers P, Topping-Morris B 1997 Clinical supervision for forensic mental health nurses. Nursing Management 4(5):13–15

Rossi K 2006 Appreciative inquiry: an overview. Online. Available at: http://www.nickheap.co.uk/articles.asp?ART_ID=211. Accessed 31/01/06

SCoR 2003a Clinical supervision framework. Society and College of Radiographers, London, UK

SCoR 2003b Clinical supervision: a position statement. Society and College of Radiographers, London, UK

Smith D 2001 Introducing clinical supervision: some pitfalls and problems. British Journal of Perioperative Nursing 11(10):436–441

Smith J 1995 Conference report – clinical supervision: conference organized by the National Health Service Executive at the National Motorcycle Museum, Solihull, 29th November 1994. Journal of Advanced Nursing 21:1029–1031

Spence C, Cantrell J, Christie I, Samet W 2002 A collaborative approach to the implementation of clinical supervision. Journal of Nursing Management 10(2):65–74

Teasdale K 2000 Practical approaches to clinical supervision. Professional Nurse 15(9):579–582

Townend M 2005 Interprofessional supervision from the perspectives of both mental health nurses and other professionals in the field of cognitive behavioural psychotherapy. Journal of Psychiatric and Mental Health Nursing 12:582–588

Watkins JM, Mohr BJ 2001 Appreciative inquiry – change at the speed of imagination. Jossey Bass Pfeiffer, San Francisco, CA, USA

Weaver M 2001 Introducing clinical supervision. British Journal of Podiatry 4(4):134–143

White E, Winstanley J 2003 Clinical supervision models and best practice. Nurse Researcher 10(4):7–38

Wilkin P, Bowers L, Monk J 1997 Clinical supervision: managing the resistance. Nursing Times 93(8):48

WMCSLS (West Midlands Clinical Supervision Learning Set) 1998 Clinical supervision: getting it right in your

organization: a critical guide to good
practice. West Midlands Clinical
Supervision Learning Set, c/o School of
Health Sciences, University of Birmingham,
UK

Wright S 1989 Changing nursing practice.
Edward Arnold, London

Wright S, Elliot M, Schofield H 1997 A
network approach to clinical supervision.
Nursing Standard 11(18):39–41

10 Setting standards for the practice of clinical supervision — a Welsh perspective

Mic Rafferty, Berwyn Llewellyn-Davies and Jeanette Hewitt

INTRODUCTION

If clinical supervision is to be truly a method of promoting, enabling and ensuring standards of care (WNB 1994), we need a means to give a form to what would count as *good* or *poor* clinical supervision practice, so that the reality of the practice of supervision can be measured against specific criteria (Rafferty et al 2003). This chapter presents a provisional standard for clinical supervision, and then draws on UK and Scandinavian literature to give practical illustrations of what practitioners and researchers have associated with each of the pre-conditions for effective clinical supervision.

The organization of the chapter describes a Provisional Standard for Clinical Supervision in Nursing and Health Visiting (Jenkins et al 2000), organized around Brigid Proctor's tripartite functions model of clinical supervision (Proctor 1986) to establish standards for practice through the use of supporting evidence. The standards were determined utilizing a modified Delphi technique, a method of tapping the knowledge, expertise or opinion of a category of people who have been defined as having specialist knowledge or expertise. The essence of the Delphi technique is that it involves repetitive surveys with a panel of experts for the purpose of developing a consensus on a specific set of topics. In this study, a panel of experienced clinical supervisors worked towards a consensus via a series of questionnaires. In the first round they were asked to write about their feelings, visual descriptions, ideas and the practical habits that they associated with their practice of clinical supervision (Rafferty et al 2003). The data were then analysed in terms of content analysis, and creation of families of resemblance, leading to concept identification and category creation. This was then circulated in the form of a standard, to the panel, for comment, leading to final modifications.

THE STANDARD STATEMENTS AS A BASELINE TO EVALUATE THE PRACTICE OF CLINICAL SUPERVISION

It is important to see the standard as provisional, and therefore open to further development and refinement, in the light of clinical supervision discoveries as to the constituents of, in a Winnicottian sense, 'good enough' clinical supervision (Rafferty 2000). The standard is useful to aid comparison with other attempts to determine performance indicators for clinical supervision. For instance, a useful bench-mark has also been developed for identifying the fundamental principles of clinical supervision and reflective practice in an organizational setting (Poulter et al 2005). Like the provisional standard, Poulter et al (2005) identify that the successful development of clinical supervision will be reliant upon its significance in the organizational agenda when understood as a key means of enabling professional development and supporting reasoned individual accountability. Driscoll (2000) in the first edition of this book points to the importance of developing mechanisms to monitor the effectiveness of clinical supervision. This is in order to create the means by which it is possible to know of the benefits or outcomes of supervision and what is good enough or not good enough practice. In this edition, the emphasis is more about using the standard as a skeleton on to which it is possible to add the developing dress code about the characteristics of good enough supervision, thereby creating the conditions from which it is realistically possible to appraise the benefits and outcomes of clinical supervision.

The standard provides a simple framework to enable practitioners and managers to engage in pragmatic negotiations about the implementation and subsequent evaluation of clinical supervision. There are nine standards that sit under three themes, namely:

- Professional support (restorative function),
- Learning from practice (formative function),
- Ensuring reasoned accountability (normative function).

The standard statements (Table 10.1) used the *structure*, *process* and *outcome* format originally developed by Donabedian (1966):

- A structure, as the name implies, offers an overall frame of reference that names the parts on which to base quality measurements in clinical supervision, rooted in the three core elements of clinical supervision described earlier.

TABLE 10.1 The provisional standards for clinical supervision

Professional Support (Restorative Function)	Time	Environment	Relationship
	Giving commitment and honouring the time for the task	Securing a venue fit for the purpose in terms of comfort, privacy, absence of interruptions	Establish a professional working relationship based on mutual trust
Learning from Practice (Formative function)	**Focus**	**Knowledge**	**Interventions**
	Attention is given to the expression of professional practice and reflection on its meaning.	Search for meaning and gathering perspectives driven by empirical knowledge and experience from practice	Affirm appropriate practice, support, professional esteem and offer achievable challenges to practice based on a secure relationship
Ensuring Accountability (Normative function)	**Organizational support**	**Recording**	**Competency**
	Provides the necessary will and resources to enable clinical supervision	An agreement is reached about the minimum content of, ownership of and access to any records kept	Use of appropriate authority and recognition of personal and professional boundaries. Support for supervisory practice and development

- The process statements, based on the available literature and experience in clinical supervision, explain, in more detail, the dynamic characteristics and what needs to happen in order to achieve the outcomes.

- The outcomes or responses indicate that satisfactory practice in clinical supervision is being achieved.

Professional supervisory relationships are ideally based on a negotiated contract and more details about this are outlined in a previous chapter by Stephen Power. In our opinion, the provisional standards also give a structure to aid negotiations about the practice of clinical supervision in order to establish the foundations for good practice. A successful outcome would be a contract that enables clinical supervision to be an opportunity for support and learning, in order to promote reasoned accountability, harm prevention, clinical development and emotional competence (Rafferty et al 2003).

WHAT WE KNOW ABOUT PROFESSIONAL SUPPORT (RESTORATIVE FUNCTIONING)

The necessary pre-conditions for professional support in clinical supervision (Table 10.1) involve judgements as to what is good enough practice in relationship to:

- appropriate *time* to do the work;
- the nature of an *environment* conducive to purpose;
- the nature of the supervisory *relationship*.

Time

Giving commitment and honouring the time for the task.

Process

Rational judgements need to be made about the necessary time required to meet emotional and developmental tasks integral to clinical supervision. Taken into account are the requirements of the clinical supervisor, supervisee and the organization.

Outcomes

We would expect that the outcomes will demonstrate that time has been made available for clinical supervision in line with rational decisions that lead to a determination of good practice.

Discussion

Time to do the work is the crucial factor in making clinical supervision a meaningful part of professional life in healthcare, without which supervision remains 'a hopeful illusory cake of possibility, rather than the bread and butter of professional life' (Thome 1999, personal communication). Therefore any attempt to propose standards for practice needs to address the significance of the time dimension. Clinical supervision has existing precedents, customs and practice in many healthcare disciplines, which show that rational judgements have been reached about what is good enough practice. Time standards exist for a number of professionals, including clinical psychologists, midwives and counsellors, for whom engagement in supervision is termed either essential or mandatory. For instance, the Chartered Society of Physiotherapy states that half a day per month should be available for 'personal learning time', including clinical supervision (CSP 2003). This notional figure of half a day per week for professional development activities is becoming an accepted norm for allied health professionals. However, for the nursing profession, making time for the activity remains a matter of choice, an exception being for those involved in child protection work in the UK, where specific child protection supervision is mandatory.

Negotiating time for what is a non-mandatory activity can be problematic. You can hear the plaintive cry of the harassed manager 'We can't even release staff for mandatory training let alone give time for clinical supervision', sometimes with an acknowledgement that it would be a good thing if only there was the time. The activity is 'endorsed and commended' by the professional regulating bodies within UK healthcare precisely because of the clear place it has in maintaining and improving standards in the often uncertain, harassed and rapidly changing health and social care environment (Gilmore 2001). Therefore it is important that time is found. Part of that process is assisting professional assertiveness about the right to have the time for clinical supervision, in what is often a time-short healthcare system and one where often instant responses are needed. This begins by identifying the continuing endorsement of clinical supervision, at the level of national strategy and local health inspectorate. For instance, numerous Department of Health documents starting with A Vision for the Future

(Department of Health 1993) identify that clinical supervision is 'central to the process of learning and the scope of professional practice'. The need to provide health professionals with time for clinical supervision is now beginning to figure more regularly in Trust reviews conducted by the Commission for Healthcare Audit and Inspection (CHAI 2004). A survey conducted by the School of Health Science, Swansea found that, for respondents offering clinical supervision, monthly sessions were the most common. However, this was qualified as the ideal standard that proved problematic for many to achieve (Rafferty et al 1998). Comments such as 'we try to ... ', '... this is our ideal' or 'if we are able' reflect the realities of squeezing sufficient time out from the unrelenting demands of the service.

Evidence suggests that the optimum time required for supervisory sessions is between 45 minutes and one and a half hours, every two to four weeks (Bond & Holland 1998, White & Winstanley 2003), with the higher frequency associated with, for example, nurses in transition after qualifying utilizing preceptorship (Jenkins et al 2000). Winstanley (2000) found that the greatest increase in positive evaluations of clinical supervision from supervisees occurred when the length of sessions was between 46 and 60 minutes. It has been suggested that the ideal frequency would be as often as once a week; however, this may be impractical given the time constraints inherent in many areas of practice (Power 1999, Severinsson & Hallberg 1996). Some authors have viewed the time dimension cynically, suggesting even world-class clinical supervision would be unlikely to be enough to help people who spend the rest of their time working in difficult environments (Wolsey & Leach 1997). Anecdotal reports from supervisees, however, counter this opinion. They suggest that the time spent in supervision is valuable time-out just for them (Bishop 1998). Clinical supervision also functions as a reference point to bring the mind and body experiences of the world of work together in order to help determine good enough responses to those demands placed on it by others (Rafferty 2000). Johns (2002:11) puts the idea of time-out from an overburdened workplace rather poetically. Reflection he says:

> ... is a state of mind, like a quiet eddy in a fast moving stream, a place to pause to consider the fast moving stream and the way the self swims within it ...

Obtain copies of your professional or organizational policies or documents relating to clinical supervision:

■ What guidance is offered or advised in relation to the amounts of time and frequency for clinical supervision?
■ Is clinical supervision a requirement within your job specification? If so, does your organization specify an optimal frequency?
■ What evidence is available to demonstrate that your organization is supportive of the practice of clinical supervision?
■ What methods do you have to monitor if clinical supervision is taking place?

On the average acute hospital ward, there may be little time available to conduct clinical supervision within a particular shift (GHNHST 2002). If supervision takes place in the worker's own time, sometimes immediately before or following the shift, then that time would need to be honoured by the organization. One hour of clinical supervision every month is equivalent to two days per year. In time-short systems such as acute medicine, these days could be added to the annual leave entitlement following negotiation with the manager. Whether an ideal state can be achieved in any sphere of health practice is debatable and it is important to consider what would be realistic and sustainable in your area and organization.

Environment

Securing a venue fit for the purpose in terms of comfort, privacy, and absence of interruptions.

Process

Finding a suitable environment for clinical supervision will be dependent on whether the methods or approaches will comprise individual activity or a group situation, held in the clinical environment or elsewhere, the available environmental resources, and organizational support. Arrangements should be made to ensure that the environment is conducive to privacy, comfort and the prevention of inappropriate distraction.

Outcome

Individuals confirm that the environment is suitable for clinical supervision. Behaviour, including non-verbal cues and verbal reports, are used to identify that the environment is appropriate, or indicate that a change of accommodation is required.

Discussion

There is evidence to show that rapport between the supervisor and supervisee is enhanced when sessions are held away from the workplace (Winstanley 2000); this may also serve to diminish the potential for guilt, for not 'caring for patients' during work time (Gilmore 2001), and there is less risk of being interrupted. However, those leaving the front line for clinical supervision in acute care may still encounter cynical remarks about indulgence or luxury (Grey 2001). Good models such as those that operate in Bro Morganwg and North Glamorgan in Wales include booking a suitable venue on a regular basis well in advance.

Where suitable environments are scarce, especially in an acute hospital setting, the use of rooms within a local educational establishment needs to be considered. Ideally, rooms should be booked six or even twelve months in advance, for booking well in advance implies a commitment to the process and mitigates against an ad-hoc approach or a 'when we can fit it in' attitude (Jenkins et al 2000). The standard process statement could be elaborated to include reference to a booking system. At the level of the ward or team, for example, a system needs to be in place where time for clinical supervision is arranged alongside off duty, annual leave and study leave. Such a system would also contribute in no small way to legitimize the activity, as it would become a concrete reality to be considered as part of the routine organization of work.

What sort of environment do you think might be suitable for your clinical supervision?

How available is it and what needs to happen for it to be used on an ongoing basis?

What might be any emotive associations with a supervision room that is used for other purposes?

How would you rate that room on a scale of 1 (poor)–5 (excellent) in Table 10.2:

TABLE 10.2

Venue	1	2	3	4	5
Privacy					
Comfort					
Distraction					
Noise					
Associations					

Relationship

Establish a professional working relationship based on mutual trust.

Process

Attention is drawn to Daniel Nichol's earlier chapter on the clinical supervision relationship and Stephen Power's chapter on the importance of contracting. Essentially, the aim is to create an egalitarian relationship, which acknowledges power differences. Rapport building is attended to by addressing issues of honesty, choice, mutual respect, sensitivity and tolerance. A relationship is created that has the potential to use uncertainty and vulnerability productively.

Outcome

Statements about emotions and congruent behaviours *from* supervisees confirm the existence of an acceptable relationship, based on values that encourage growth. If the relationship is unacceptable within the clinical supervision process appropriate action is taken.

Discussion

Effective clinical supervision will stand or fall on the supervisory relationship and the quality of the mutual and working alliance established (Proctor 1986). The quality of the relationship has primacy of effect over any model or theory employed to understand human experience, guide interventions or judge outcomes (Bambling & King 2001). Importantly, having a poor clinical supervisor may do more harm than having no supervisor at all. Inappropriate and unskilled practice may result in feelings of isolation and guilt in the supervisee (Burnard 1990). Poor relationships may lead to unethical violations of confidentiality, a breakdown of professional and personal boundaries or less than respectful treatment of the supervisee (West 2003). It needs to be kept in mind that a sense of vulnerability in the supervisee is not uncommon in the early stages of the clinical supervisory relationship (Johns 2003). This element of the standard requires that attention be paid to creating an egalitarian alliance or a co-operative alliance (Proctor 2001). Understanding and acknowledging power differences within the supervisory relationship is an important factor in building such an alliance.

Consider how the different types of power, as described by French and Raven (1968), can enhance or threaten the clinical supervision relationship and what agreements will need to be made with your clinical supervisor beforehand to counter the following:
- The clinical supervisor has the ability and resources to obtain rewards for those who comply with directives.
- The clinical supervisor exercises influence because of perceived attractiveness, reputation or charisma.
- The clinical supervisor has the ability to punish undesirable outcomes.
- The clinical supervisor is someone who is competent and who has some specialist knowledge or expertise in a given area.
- The clinical supervisor has a right and authority to exercise influence because of a leadership role or position in the organization.
- What questions might you ask a potential clinical supervisor to ensure that your clinical supervisory relationship gets off to a positive start?

Valued personal characteristics of the supervisor have been identified as warmth, empathy, humour and caring (Simms 1993). The qualities of genuineness, empathy, being non-judgemental and able to listen actively are positive characteristics of an effective clinical supervisor (Butterworth 1992; Devine & Baxter 1995). The supervisor should be able to develop supportive relationships, through being perceptive to the supervisee's needs, and being able to give and receive constructive criticism. Winstanley (2000) also linked the idea of choice to a positive outcome for the supervisory relationship. Thus, honesty, mutual respect, sensitivity and tolerance, central to a person-centred relationship, are the values most readily associated with a professional relationship likely to encourage personal and professional growth (Sloan 1998).

From the point of view of someone seeking clinical supervision it is important to think seriously about what you want or need from clinical supervision. Those new and inexperienced will have different needs to some of us who are, shall we say, more long-in-the-tooth. The clinical supervisor and supervisee need to consider whether the experience is available to recognize and meet the needs of different professional transitions and challenges.

If the supervisor displays person-centred qualities or conditions consistently over time then, according to Carl Rogers, the relationship has the foundation to allow for growth and change to take place (Rogers 1962). Utilizing the ideas of Bowlby about attachment theory, Cottrell (2004) investigated the qualities of a clinical supervisor that were required to promote growth. Cottrell suggests that good enough supervisors are secure, insightful and consistent with a capacity for empathy. They are able to support and challenge appropriately, pay attention to their own emotions and have an affiliative working style. Importantly they can attend to both relationship and task issues in clinical supervision at the same time.

Healthcare professionals often cope directly with human suffering in daily practice and may develop defence mechanisms to deal with the distress of caring. This may lead the worker to be distant from the patient or, conversely, to over-involvement (Jones 1997). Therefore it is necessary for the supervisor to possess the quality of empathy in order to sensitively draw into awareness attitudes which may be adversely affecting caring relationships. The supervisor must also have the ability to tolerate and work with the attendant anxiety evoked by such personal insights and hold the supervisee through periods of uncertainty and associated vulnerability.

It is important that those engaged in clinical supervision are able to articulate how this egalitarian relationship contributes to an outcome of personal and professional growth. This is especially so when faced with tokenistic attitudes towards implementation.

Operational expediency may ignore the importance of choice and the time needed for relationship building. This may lead to supervisory arrangements that are orientated towards outcomes rather than the quality of the process (e.g. overconcerned with clinical and managerial task completion rather than a professional's care work experience).

As identified in the standard, in supervisory relationships, supervisees need to feel safe enough to evaluate whether the relationship is working or not. The intention to engage in periodic evaluation of the relationship should then form part of the initial contract.

WHAT WE KNOW ABOUT LEARNING FROM PRACTICE (FORMATIVE FUNCTIONING)

The second group of standards is about *learning*. Clinical practice learning involves attention to a practice *focus*, through the use of relevant *knowledge* and supervisory *interventions*. Through the medium of guided reflection, clinical supervision enables clinicians to develop clinical practice and supports continuous learning, reducing the risk of errors and poor practices (Wilkin et al 1997, Wright et al 1997). It is also a means of promoting quality of patient care in a dynamic and innovative way, through meeting the personal and professional needs of health professionals faced with the task of adapting to the constantly changing facets of professional life and practice (Barber & Norman 1987, Gilmore 2001, Snow & Willard 1989, UKCC 1996). These elements of learning express the primary purpose of clinical supervision — to improve care through critical appraisal of practice experiences (Jenkins et al 2000).

Focus

Attention is given to the expression of professional practice and reflection on its meaning.

Process

The focus of clinical supervision is the supervisee's expression of their professional practice, including the experience of supervision, and reflection upon its meanings.

Outcome

Accounts about supervision, provided by the supervisee and supervisor, identify that practice and its professional and personal meaning is the focus.

Discussion

The focus of clinical supervision is to reflect on the supervisee's work process, responding to the unfolding situations that present within everyday practice. It is a structured method of exploring practice: to make judgements on past and future practices, to inform better future actions. At the heart of healthcare is the practice of human concern and this tends to flourish if workers are provided with opportunities to talk about their work. This opportunity to talk can attend to different levels of professional insight and maturity. For instance, Hawkins and Shohet (2000) describe a developmental approach within clinical supervision. A supervisee at the outset of their career may want to focus on the question of the practicalities of work: 'How do I do my job and what are the options?' At an advanced level of functioning, where the supervisory relationship is firmly established, the question is 'Who am I in my job and how do arrive at my judgements?' At both ends of this continuum of the focus of clinical supervision is the necessity to address the uncertainties of practice, ever present for both the novice and the expert.

For both novice and expert, work is meaningful because it parallels the worker's experience of living the life to its natural conclusion and that leads to the formation of values that, in turn, inform the care given. The implication of this for the practitioner is that they are faced continually with the meaning of 'what it is to be' in order to arrive at new judgements about themselves and the effectiveness of their practice. Whatever the level of experience, the focus of clinical supervision must reflect on the most mundane to the most complex aspects of work, because nothing should be taken for granted but always viewed with an open and curious mind (Johns 2002).

Gordon and Benner (1980) provide a helpful framework to capture the nature of professional life in its naturalness. They explored the nature of expert practice, by encouraging nurses to talk about their work in terms of what they did that really made a difference to patients or give an example of a practice event that went unusually well. In addition, to capture the complete gambit of usual practice, they encouraged nurses to explore an incident where there was a breakdown, when things did not go so well or where practice was particularly demanding. Respondents also talked about events in practice that they regarded as ordinary or typical which captured the quintessential nature of their practice. Such a frame of reference is a useful starting point to help you to consider what can be the focus of clinical supervision.

A question arises as to what level of attention upon the internal personal world of the professional can be legitimately focused on in clinical supervision. Heath and Freshwater (2000) suggest that we have much to learn about how to work with such matters, given the inevitable vulnerability this engenders, compounded by the potential for illegitimate intrusion into personal matters. A safe starting point is for the supervisee to decide what level of enquiry would be right for them. Hicks and Samuels (2002) recommend a pre-contract meeting with perhaps more than one potential clinical supervisor. Here the supervisee asks a prepared series of questions to ascertain the style and anticipated content of supervision from the perspective supervisor and, above all, to gain a sense of compatibility of the working alliance. As Proctor (2001) identifies, clinical supervision evolves into different forms depending on the needs of the individual and the supervisor. Therefore, it is important for the supervisee to have self-conscious control of what they want from the process and be able to check this out with the potential supervisor before committing themselves. Thus, adequate preparation for clinical supervision is vital, because participants need to enter this process with their eyes wide open. When clinical supervision is working effectively it offers unique opportunities for practice to be both challenged and supported.

The formal structure of clinical supervision purposefully examines both the *theory to practice* and *practice to theory* links that other informal supportive staff networks would not necessarily do. This is because sessions are structured toward an outcome: the devising of an action plan intended to have a direct and practical impact on practice that is later reviewed for its effectiveness. Thus *good enough* clinical supervision impacts on practice for the benefit of the patient. Anecdotal and experiential evidence suggests clinical supervision provides health professionals with the means to access the lived experience of practice via a rich narrative. The good news is that such narratives confirm that, by and large, we have a healthcare workforce who can demonstrate concerned artistry in the practice of their profession.

Because of practice audit, detail is becoming available about what is brought to sessions by clinical supervisees. Thinking about your own practice situations over the past months, how familiar are the following themes identified by Pugsley and Edwards (2003) as possibilities for your own clinical supervision? What might you add to the list?

- Situations in the clinical setting.
- Aggression and violence in the workplace.
- Management issues.
- Staff relationships.
- New legislation.
- Training and education.
- Other?

Knowledge

Search for meaning and gathering perspectives driven by empirical knowledge and experience from practice.

Process

The issue of knowledge in clinical supervision is complex, as it concerns the understanding of people, and therefore of human dynamics. Knowledge about human dynamics is available on at least two levels. Firstly, knowledge that is brought to the clinical supervision represents best practice, e.g. empirical knowledge (what is known) and, equally importantly, revealed knowledge that arises out of the study of practice known as local practice theory. Therefore, clinical supervision is a medium for the study of relationship dynamics, central to healthcare work, as it allows the integration of theory with practice and the articulation of practice, which leads to the generation of the theory.

Outcome

Accounts about supervision provided by the supervisee and supervisor acknowledge degrees of professional and emotional competence and identify the dynamic nature of learning.

Discussion

To understand the relationship dynamics of healthcare it is often proposed that the clinical supervisor should be an experienced practitioner who has an understanding of the issues relevant to the supervisee's practice (Butterworth & Faugier 1992, Kohner 1994, Power 1999, UKCC 1996). However, clinical experience does not necessarily equal excellence as a clinical supervisor, as the kinds of clinical supervision skills wanted are not readily transferable from many other areas of supervision practice. Therefore it may be more important to focus on the primacy of supervisory skills and not necessarily the professional experience of the supervisor (Kohner 1994, Nicklin 1997). As a generalization, it may be argued that the expert practitioner, by overlaying their own experience onto the issue brought to clinical supervision, may be more directive than facilitative in their learning approach to the supervisee. The practitioner, therefore, is not encouraged to step back to consider the efficacy and appropriateness of their interventions practised during the delivery of care (Jones 1997). The power asymmetry in clinical supervision means that the supervisee may accept the expert practitioner status of the supervisor and their interpretation of events uncritically (Jones 1997). A degree of courage is another quality to be added to the necessary mix for exploring one's attitude practices when working in healthcare, because to do this inevitably means making sense of the personal responses to human conflict and distress (Rafferty 1998). However, there is a choice as to how one deals with such exposure; either it can be used as a source of learning (and lead to the challenges of exploring unknown territory) or the feelings evoked can be ignored or suppressed (for the sake of an easier life and not succumbing to the perceived 'weakness' of having a need for clinical supervision).

The notion of reflective learning is central to clinical supervision, and as several authors advise (Johns 1993, Kohner 1994, Saylor 1990), effective reflection does not occur spontaneously and is a learnt ability. The qualities necessary for such learning have been described by Johns (2002) as:

- Intelligence: a disposition to alter beliefs.
- Curiosity: an ability to seek out information.
- Reflectiveness: an ability to evaluate own beliefs.
- Wilfulness: an ability to act on one's reflections.

Such ideas are helpful to both the supervisee and supervisor, when thinking about learning outcomes that inform the work. The role of the clinical supervisor is to guide reflection-on-practice. This is not a skill that can be taught just formally; rather, the facilitation skills necessary to enable this process are more effectively attained through experiential learning with others (Butterworth & Faugier 1992, Hawkins & Shohet 2000). Johns (1993) has given guidance using Schon's model (1987) of reflection on and in action, but it is equally important to recognize the place of anticipatory reflection (Greenwood 1993). Johns identified the format of setting the scene, then reflecting on, or anticipating (Greenwood, 1993) the event, identifying alternative actions and determining what learning has taken place. Reflection-on-practice is not an unfamiliar idea to healthcare professionals, in that they have always done it through story telling (Wolsey & Leach 1997). However, while clinicians may have always told the stories of care they have not always self-consciously learned from them.

The value of reflection is that it allows the supervisee to learn from their caring art. Healthcare practitioners require skills that allow them to make immediate responses to complex situations. Most of the decisions required on a daily basis find their solutions not in textbooks but out of the reasoning of experience. The problem is that this reasoning of experience is usually outside self-conscious awareness. Clinical supervision, as a vehicle for guided reflection, provides an opportunity for the practitioner to draw into awareness their complex array of enabling and helping skills, revealed in everyday actions, leading to more self-conscious reflection in action (Schon 1987) and reflection before action (Greenwood 1993). Therefore the practice of guided reflection aids the development of the 'internal supervisor' and the habit of self-observation (Casement 1990, Jones 1997).

We know from pre-registration educational experience that evaluating whether progressive learning has taken place can be done through the assessment of written portfolios. The usual model adopted has an agreed model for reflection, with the student or supervisee encouraged to write about critical incidents, going on to identify and critically analyse thoughts, feelings and behaviour before, during, and after the incident. The aim of these exercises is to promote increased self-awareness and to identify deficits and strengths in knowledge and skills. Where deficits are identified the supervisee may also use the portfolio to explore and document new knowledge of evidence-based practice to enhance future management of similar incidents. Growth thus can be measured through examination and discussion of the portfolio. While this is applicable for an education setting it is less likely to be the case in clinical supervision.

- In what ways might professional learning be identified through clinical supervision?
- How might this be evidenced to others working in clinical practice?

Interventions

Affirm appropriate practice, support professional esteem and offer achievable challenges to practice based on a secure relationship.

Process

Interventions affirm appropriate practice, and support personal and professional esteem and the search for developmentally achievable professional challenges.

Outcome

Feedback about supervision provided by the supervisee and supervisor includes reports about increased wellbeing and plans of action to utilize professional competence and meet learning needs.

Discussion

Hawkins and Shohet (2000) describe different types of intervention within clinical supervision. Firstly, there is the focus on what was happening between the health professional and patient. This involves:

- Looking at factors concerning the content of the situation — what was said and perhaps not said, what was done, and in what order.
- Looking at options — what was chosen and why, what alternatives were available.
- Looking at the situation from a different angle.

While this might give a surface approach to what is spoken about in clinical supervision, psychodynamic theory focuses on the dynamics that may unfold between the supervisee and the supervisor as also being part of intervening in clinical supervision. These may be subtle and some exploration may be necessary to bring them to conscious awareness. This acts as a means of raising the awareness of the supervisee about what may be happening in the practice situation.

The sorts of ways interventions can be discovered in clinical supervision can be through reflecting on the feelings of the supervisee, evoked by the patient or practice situation. An example is given by Mattinson (1975), who discusses the importance of having an awareness of the psychological distance that may exist at certain times between the practitioner and the patient, which can exert an influence on the quality of care both given and received. One important task within clinical supervision is to then explore the question of 'What did this patient make me feel like?' Insights gained from reflecting in this way could then be taken back to benefit practice. Attending to non-verbal cues and changes in the demeanour of the supervisee in the supervision session may mirror what is happening (unconsciously) in the practice situation and is a further way of understanding interventions between the supervisee and the client/patient. Jones (1997) illustrates how a nurse absorbed a patient's hidden distress and mirrored this unconsciously in the supervisory relationship. In this sense, clinical supervision gave calm and order to painful emotions and strong feelings near the surface were uncovered and explored in safety. In a later study, Jones (1998) reported that conflicts in practice and not just the patient can then also be mirrored in the supervisory encounter. Often a supervisor can simply be intuitive to their own feelings that the supervisee rouses in clinical supervision rather than relying on what is verbalized. Benner (1984) argues that the expert practitioner, with a wealth of experience and an intuitive grasp of each situation, zeros in on the problem without wasteful consideration of a large range of alternative diagnoses and solutions. In the same way, the experienced supervisor may have an intuitive grasp of, and response to, a situation in supervision that is not easily articulated or explained.

Further ideas about psychological intervention skills that can be used in clinical supervision can also be found in the previous chapter by Graham Sloan. Much will depend on the interpersonal skills of the supervisor and willingness of the supervisee to accept such interventions as being part of clinical supervision. Rafferty (2000) argues that having a supervisory ability to challenge practice blind spots, being able to 'hold' the expression of emotion and enable free expression, are interventions that are at the heart of clinical supervision.

WHAT WE KNOW ABOUT PROFESSIONAL ACCOUNTABILITY (NORMATIVE FUNCTIONING)

The third element of the standard concerns professional accountability and includes organizational and personal accountability through the establishment of systems to communicate information and monitor the competence of supervisory practice.

Organizational support

Provides the necessary will and resources to enable clinical supervision.

Process

The organization provides the necessary will and resources to enable supervisees and supervisors to respectively receive or offer appropriate clinical supervision.

Outcome

Organizational monitoring identifies the patterns of supervisory practice and their match with strategic direction and resources.

Discussion

The successful implementation of clinical supervision in healthcare settings can be judged on the degree to which the activity is embedded in the culture of the workplace. Organizational support and active sponsorship are essential to the enterprise. Historically individual health professionals have championed the cause to take forward clinical supervision, with the result of its implementation often being described as patchy or in pockets. When it is just 'another thing to do' that adds to an overburdened workload, the prospects of successful implementation are remote. Clinical supervision provides an important means for health organizations to invest in and recognize the quality of staff. Maybe the question that needs to be addressed is not how to implement clinical supervision in isolation, posed in the previous chapter, but how an organization can best support its staff. Through a culture, which is supportive of its staff, clinical supervision should be embraced as a norm rather than an exception.

For change to take place certain factors need to operate in tandem. Consider how your work setting is equipped to embrace the process of change to incorporate clinical supervision into the working culture, for example:

- Is there a shared vision?
- Are people prepared adequately in terms of awareness and skills?
- What incentives are there for people to engage in the process?
- What resources are available (e.g. time, a suitable venue)?
- Is there a plan of action?
- Are there plans to monitor, audit and evaluate the process?
- What will be some of the differences between your own vision of being involved in clinical supervision and that of the organization?

For organizations to invest in clinical supervision they need to be satisfied that there will be tangible and measurable improvements in services. Mechanisms for monitoring effectiveness and outcomes can be used to justify clinical supervisory time and maintaining agreed levels of competency (Burrow 1995). At the same time, organizational structures need to be in place whereby the benefits of clinical supervision can be articulated and communicated at the corporate level. Another advantage to the organization is that clinical supervision acts as a barometer of the workplace. What is needed is a process whereby themes from practice can be communicated to the appropriate level to influence organizational learning.

Evaluation is also needed to assess how clinical supervision can influence care (UKCC 1996). This may be achieved through a mixture of qualitative and quantitative methods to observe changes in clinical practice. Organizations would be interested in, for example, auditing and monitoring sickness/absence rates before and after the introduction of clinical supervision. Other methods might include monitoring staff satisfaction scales, the number and nature of complaints, retention and recruitment of staff, career progression and critical incident maps (Butterworth & Bishop 1996; Marrow et al 1998). Caution is to be exercised in relationship to such production line objectives for clinical supervision (Heath & Freshwater 2000), as they are generally only responsive to macro organizational morale (Main 1989) and not necessarily to what happens in clinical supervision. Whether there is a truth in such claims will only be answered when there is a considerable critical mass of participants, allowing evaluation.

The clinical supervision evaluation project (Butterworth et al 1997) reported on the effects of clinical supervision on nurses. Results from the study accumulated data on levels of stress, job satisfaction and psychological wellbeing from 586 nurses engaged in clinical supervision. There was some evidence that staff felt supported and protected by the process. Teasdale and associates (2001) carried out a study that described and measured the effects of clinical supervision on

211 qualified nurses. This study found that those receiving clinical supervision had a more positive experience of management, showed increased coping skills and perceived that they were in receipt of greater levels of support, particularly at a junior level. Drawing on Butterworth's work, the Clinical Supervision Evaluation Project (Winstanley 2000) has developed the Manchester clinical supervision scale (MCSS), which evaluates clinical supervision on seven dimensions. Use of the MCSS revealed evidence to uphold the view that nurses experience personal support for their practice as a result of receiving clinical supervision. The quality of clinical supervision was shown to be dependent on factors external to the supervisory relationship, including the organizational and managerial culture (Winstanley & White 2003). However, little could be gleaned about the effects on patient care and this remains the Holy Grail for clinical supervision research.

The establishment of clinical governance in UK healthcare is a major driver for those who advocate an organizational approach to the implementation of clinical supervision. Greater emphasis in the healthcare agenda is upon the issues of quality and public safety. It has raised their importance to equal that of financial concerns. Clinical governance is defined as:

> A framework through which NHS organizations are accountable for continuously improving the quality of services and safeguarding high standards of care, by creating an environment in which excellence in clinical care will flourish. Department of Health, 1979

It places importance on corporate and individual accountability and the continuous development of care. Some of the broad principles underpinning clinical governance in UK healthcare include:

- Leadership and accountability.
- Continuing quality improvement.
- Continuing professional development.
- Risk management/managing poor performance.

Clinical supervision not only complements these principles but has the potential to act as a foundation from which the clinical governance agenda can thrive in the clinical area in so far as it is seen as a mechanism that is supportive of practitioners in their delivery of care. The implementation of clinical supervision in Wales using clinical governance is an ongoing process. You might wish to read some of the steps being taken to ensure organizational support for clinical supervision.

Representatives from a wide range of stakeholders, including the Welsh Assembly, NHS trusts, education establishments and the independent sector, have been meeting to consider the current state of clinical supervision in Wales and to make recommendations as to how to take it forward (All Wales Clinical Supervision Group 2004–2005). These discussions informed a clinical supervision implementation project in Gwent Healthcare Trust. A four-year investment was made to create an infrastructure to train and support clinical supervisors, legitimize the practice of clinical supervision and develop systems whereby the benefits of clinical supervision are articulated and themes from practice inform organizational learning.

A full time project co-ordinator was seconded to work in conjunction with a steering group made up of senior managers representing all the divisions within the Trust. The project operated on the person-centred principles of choice, trust and ownership. Emphasis was given to addressing the question of how an organization could best support its staff, with the offer of clinical supervision as a supportive mechanism. The Trust's position is that everyone should be given the opportunity to access clinical supervision if they so choose. Managers and practitioners are responsible for thinking creatively about organizing appropriate time, identifying suitable environments and, importantly, developing a system to enable sessions to be booked well in advance.

Clinical supervision is a skilled activity. Those accessing clinical supervision must be guaranteed an appropriate standard of service. A baseline assessment revealed a skill deficit to fulfil the role of clinical supervisor. A training programme was necessary to meet this need. An in-house programme was implemented as it afforded flexibility in its delivery and could cater for the number of participants involved. It was delivered over twelve two-hour sessions in closed groups of four with a facilitator. The aims were to ensure a measurable standard of practice and build the capacity of clinical supervisors. It also provided the basis for evaluating the impact of clinical supervision. A longitudinal research proposal has been developed, currently in its pilot stage, to evaluate the effectiveness of clinical supervision for individuals. An ambitious second phase of the research project aims to develop a methodology to measure the effects of clinical supervision on practice.

The main engine to drive clinical supervision forward on a sustainable basis is the clinical supervisors' forum. Its functions are threefold:

- to provide peer support for clinical supervisors' practice,
- to develop knowledge and skills via keynote presentations and discussion, and
- manage processes such as audit and the maintenance of standards and competency.

An important task for members of the forum is to identify and anonymize themes from practice, and present them at a corporate level to inform organizational learning. By acknowledging the role of clinical supervisor and their representation at corporate level the organization makes visible its commitment to legitimize the process. In return there is need for evidence of the added value of clinical supervision for the number of hours invested.

More detailed approaches to clinical supervision can be found in the previous chapter. However, developing a culture (and organizational support) for clinical supervision remains as slow and ongoing a process across Wales as we suspect anywhere else. The value of clinical supervision needs to be articulated in terms of how it benefits the practitioner, patient and, not least, the organization. The task facing the current stakeholders and, importantly, future generations across Wales is adequate preparation (in terms of organizational infrastructure and training) in order to embed the activity as routine best practice.

Recording

An agreement is reached about the minimum content, ownership and access to any record kept.

Process

Supervisees, supervisors and the organization responsibly negotiate models of supervisee-held records that specify minimum content and the conditions for access determined.

Outcome

Contracts drawn up between supervisor and supervisee are specific in the agreement on record keeping.

Discussion

Just as the supervisory relationship should be fundamentally honest and transparent, so the methods by which information is recorded and stored should be similarly transparent. Information and reporting to managers and other departments should be clear, both in the content of such information and the processes by which it is delivered. Lack of clarity in this area can lead to concealment of important issues on both an organizational and an individual level. Aspects of record keeping form part of the contact between the supervisor and the supervisee and should detail content, ownership, access and storage. It is generally advised that the supervisee take responsibility for record keeping unless clinical supervision is a requirement of the employee's contract, in which case it will be the property of the employer (UKCC 1992). Although it rarely happens, records of clinical supervision may have to be disclosed in a court of law. In the criminal court and industrial tribunal, records can be subpoenaed and in the civil court there is a duty to disclose the records, whoever owns them (RCN 1999). Brigit Dimond (1998) has even suggested that the wisdom of keeping records in clinical supervision is questionable.

■ What records do you or would you consider keeping of your sessions in clinical supervision and why?
■ What might be some of the advantages and disadvantages of keeping records in clinical supervision and why?
■ Obtain and read the following article: Cutcliffe J 2000 To record or not record: documentation in clinical supervision. British Journal of Nursing 9(6):350–355.
■ How does this leave you now in relation to record keeping in clinical supervision?
■ What advice does your professional organization give about record keeping in clinical supervision?

Clinical supervision records can provide a structure for reflection as well as be an *aide-mémoire* to help the supervisee to focus on the salient points of the discussion and provide evidence of development in practice. However, periodic review of documentation and records of parties engaged in clinical supervision can either be positively regarded as evidence validating the learning and growth of the practitioner or be negatively viewed as a form of intrusion and surveillance of health professionals by the organization. This latter negative view might impede the implementation of clinical supervision.

Competency

Use of appropriate authority and recognition of personal and professional boundaries. Support for supervisory practice and development.

Process

Competent supervisory practice requires the use of appropriate authority and the recognition of personal and professional boundaries.

Outcome

Supervisors' supervision ensures that the exercise of authority and maintenance of personal and professional boundaries is appropriate.

Discussion

As identified by the UKCC position paper (1996), the preparation of supervisors is crucial to the success of clinical supervision. Since then, the Nursing and Midwifery Council (which replaced the UKCC) and other health professional bodies (COT 1997, CSP 2005 NMC 2005, SCoR 2003) have placed emphasis upon the importance of 'relevant practice experience'. It has been found that ongoing experiential learning and training in supervisory practice is the principal means of developing supervisory competence: the development of the necessary skills, qualities and characteristics (listening, facilitating constructive reflection and the ability to guide practitioners to appropriate outcomes) depends on practice. Arguably, if staff have a greater awareness of the nature of clinical supervision then they will be more likely to participate in receiving and providing the service. Thus, competency begins with raising awareness for all staff within an organization during induction into employment.

In the main, clinical supervision is introduced during specialist post-registration courses, so the development of clinical supervisory skills and an understanding of the value of clinical supervision is being achieved with only a minority of practitioners in Wales. At present pre-registration students are replete with the skills of self-reflective practice but to maintain and develop those skills as supervisors in the future workplace requires the ability to facilitate the reflections of others. The call must be for curriculum re-design (Cutcliffe 2001) to include supervisory skills training so that, on entering the realities of practice, newly qualified staff will be better able to offer support for reflective practice on a routine basis.

All registered healthcare professionals need to know in detail what clinical supervision is in order to be able to make an informed choice about adopting it as a part of professional practice. Preparation workshops of one or two days' duration can provide enough baseline knowledge and insights into this experiential process to equip the practitioner for the role of 'novice' clinical supervisee or supervisor. It is important that initial preparatory workshops emphasize that the development of skills is not only of benefit to supervisors but also to the benefit of their future supervisees. However, surveys reveal that without further support following preparatory workshops the activity is more than likely to cease due to the lack of confidence and competence (DCNHST 2003, GNHST 2002).

Health professionals who wish to develop further as clinical supervisors and receive preparation about how to introduce clinical supervision into practice have opportunities to enrol on clinical supervision modules. However, the numbers of health professionals interested in pursuing this academic route are few, relative to the service need. There is a case for organizations to develop the Open College or National Vocational Qualification (NVQ) route to awards. There are certain advantages in that it is a cost-effective way to provide a framework for basic preparation delivered in-house and it is attractive to clinicians who gain from experiential learning and who do not wish to engage in advanced academic courses. Running courses in-house will also raise the profile of clinical supervision and encourage further participation.

Advanced practitioner awards, at BSc and MSc level, are however essential for the future development of the practice of clinical supervision in healthcare. At present, the knowledge base in healthcare (as opposed to other disciplines) in the current educational provision is underdeveloped. More work is needed to develop competencies and explanations about clinical supervision practice in healthcare from a specific theoretical orientation (e.g. psychodynamic, systemic, cognitive, humanistic, and group explanations).

- What training is available for clinical supervision within your area?
- How has this provision (if you have had any) equipped you with the confidence to then offer a service as a clinical supervisor?
- As a supervisee what questions would you ask a potential supervisor to be assured of their competence?

The standard pays attention to important issues concerning the practice of clinical supervisors, for instance drawing attention to the fact that the role requires the exercise of appropriate authority and the recognition of personal and professional boundaries. It suggests that the monitoring of the supervisors' ability to meet such requirements would be best served by supervisors having their practice as clinical supervisors supervised.

There is the potential for an abusive or collusive relationship to develop within the supervisee–supervisor relationship. While there are no reports of such patterns of supervisory abuse in health disciplines, the lessons learnt by the discipline of counselling suggest there needs to be an explicit system to deal with complaints. These can be extrapolated from the various codes of professional conduct for health practitioners. For many, reasonable conditions of safe practice of supervision have been established. Practice models show that it is possible to develop such oversight structures in-house, or within a consultancy arrangement with an educational provider. It is important to note that the emphasis within such forums is upon developing competence in being supportive and enabling and not in surveillance.

CONCLUSION

The intention of this chapter was to describe a provisional standard for clinical supervision (Table 10.1) that used a functions approach to suggest key issues and tasks for consideration when adopting clinical supervision in healthcare practice. Development of the standard for clinical supervision has been used to also assemble the literature to state what is known about the necessary practice conditions for good and therefore more probably effective clinical supervision. The issues addressed in this chapter are perhaps the most important issues in this book as they take you beyond rhetoric about clinical supervision towards your future practice of clinical supervision.

Clinical or, perhaps more accurately, practice supervision is an important development in fostering professional self-regulation by peers. No better mechanism is apparent for developing thoughtful and mindful care by the effective study of practice that in turn can lead to the development of practice theory (Dickoff et al 1968). Health professionals, because of clinical supervision, have assured and available peer support to better make sense of the joys and sorrows of the practice of professional concern.

Conversely, clinical supervision also has the potential to be yet one other means to control and dis-emancipate health professionals (Maggs 1998) through lip service, overemphasizing normative managerial agendas and poor supervision practice. The health professional in such cases can reasonably argue that a duty of care has not been met. Therefore, it is important to begin to articulate perspectives about the 'good enough' practice of clinical supervision which establishes baselines.

The key issues and tasks identified in the standard provide guidance about what is becoming to be regarded as the necessary process of clinical supervision (in terms of time for effectiveness, the nature of thoughtful environments and helpful and harmless professional relationships) that provides mutual support and restoration. Mapping out the focus, the nature of pertinent knowledge and some of the strategies useful for clinical supervision points to its importance in professional life. Through attention to both the *taken for granted* and *exceptional practice* experiences the health professional is able to get a fresh sense of a practice experience, with all this implies in terms of impact on attitudes, values, philosophy, knowledge and practice. It is important therefore to know more about the interventions that constitute good enough clinical supervision. The standard's attention to focus, knowledge and interventions provides a conceptually stable framework to guide future evaluation and research about the point of clinical supervision in professional life.

The normative function establishes the strategic responsibility of healthcare organizations to support professional supervision practice and gives tangible illustrations of what this means in terms of necessary resources and processes. The standard provides a sensible way forward about the contentious issue of recording, which cannot be dodged, because one of the responsibilities of professional practice is to establish a narrative about the trivia, trials and triumphs of that practice, in support of reasoned accountability and clinical governance. It is becoming increasingly apparent that clinical supervision is a practice, rather more than just a set of skills, with health professionals as clinical supervisors and supervisees requiring preparation rather than training. The chapter illustrates innovative approaches to preparation that make it more likely that supervisor–supervisee development will be regarded as a lifelong adventure, providing considerable opportunities for research into the experience of supervision and establishing its relationship to good care.

In conclusion, clinical supervision still requires judgements about what is good practice in relation to:

- time, environment and relationship,
- focus, knowledge and intervention,
- organizational support, recording and competency.

We would welcome continuing this dialogue with you and your colleagues.

REFERENCES

Bambling M, King R 2001 The therapeutic alliance and clinical practice. Psychotherapy in Australia 8(1):38–43

Barber P, Norman I 1987 Skills in supervision. Nursing Times 80(2):3

Benner P 1984 From novice to expert: excellence and power in clinical nursing practice. Addison-Wesley, Menlo Park, California

Bishop V 1998 Clinical supervision: what's going on? Results of a questionnaire. Nursing Times 94(18):50–53

Bond M, Holland S 1998 Skills of clinical supervision for nurses. Open University, Buckingham

Burnard P 1990 Learning human skills: an experiential guide for nurses. 2nd edn. Butterworth-Heinemann, London

Burrow S 1995 Supervision: clinical development or management control? British Journal of Nursing 4(15):879–882

Butterworth T 1992 Clinical supervision as an emerging idea in nursing. In: Butterworth T, Faugier J (eds) Clinical supervision and mentorship in nursing. Chapman and Hall, London

Butterworth TV, Bishop 1996 First steps towards evaluating clinical supervision in nursing and health visiting: 1 theory, policy and practice development. A review. Journal of Clinical Nursing 5(2):127–132

Butterworth TJ, Carson et al 1997 It is good to talk. The University of Manchester, Manchester

Butterworth T, Faugier J (eds) 1992 Clinical supervision and mentorship in nursing. Chapman and Hall, London

Casement P 1990 Further learning from the patient: the analytic space and process. Tavistock/Routledge, London

CHAI 2004 Cambridgeshire and Peterborough Mental Health Partnership NHS Trust clinical governance review (May). Commission for Healthcare Audit and Inspection. Online. Available at: www.chai.org.uk/assetRoot/04/00/17/56/0 4001756.pdf. Accessed 18/09/05

COT 1997 Statement on supervision in occupational therapy SPP 150(A). College of Occupational Therapists, London

Cottrell S 2004 The influence on attachment style on clinical supervision style in nurses and allied professions. Unpublished MPhil thesis, University of Bangor

CSP 2003 Continuing professional development (CPD). Briefing and policy statement. Chartered Society of Physiotherapy, London, UK (July)

CSP 2005 A guide to implementing clinical supervision (information paper: CPD 37). The Chartered Society of Physiotherapy, London, UK

Cutcliffe J 2001 An alternative training approach in clinical supervision. In: Cutcliffe J, Butterworth T, Proctor B (eds) Fundamental themes in clinical supervision. Routledge, London, UK, p 47–63

DCNHST 2003 Clinical supervision. A staff survey. Denbighshire and Conway NHS Trust, Wales

Department of Health 1993 A vision for the future. National Health Service Management Executive, HMSO, London

Department of Health 1999 Clinical governance: quality in the new NHS. DOH, Leeds, UK

Devine A, Baxter D 1995 Introducing clinical supervision: a guide. Nursing Standard 9(40):32–34

Dickoff J, James P 1968 A theory of theories: a position paper. Nursing Research 17(3):197–203

Dimond B 1998 Legal aspects of clinical supervision 1: employer vs. employee. British Journal of Nursing 7(7):393–395

Donabedian A 1966 Quality of care: problems of measurement, part II. Some issues of evaluating the quality of nursing care. American Journal of Public Health 59:1833–1836

Driscoll J 2000 Practising clinical supervision: a reflective approach. Baillière Tindall, Edinburgh

French J, Raven B 1968 The bases of social power. In: Cartwright D, Zander A (eds) Group dynamics. Row Peterson, Evanston, IL, p 150–167

GHNHST 2002 Clinical supervision: a staff survey. Gwent Healthcare NHS Trust, Wales

Gilmore A 2001 Clinical supervision in nursing and health visiting: a review of the literature. In: Cutcliffe J, Butterworth T, Proctor B (eds) Fundamental themes in clinical supervision. London, Routledge, p 125–140

Gordon D, Benner P 1980 Guidelines for recording critical incidents The AMICAE project University of San Francisco. In: Benner P (ed) Novice to expert. Addison Wesley, Menlo Park, CA

Greenwood J 1993 Reflective practice: a critique of the work of Argyris and Schon. Journal of Advanced Nursing 19:1183–1187

Grey W 2001 Conducting clinical and managerial supervision. Nursing Management 3(6):14–22

Hawkins P, Shohet R 2000 Supervision in the helping professions. Open University, Milton Keynes

Heath H, Freshwater D 2000 Clinical supervision as an emancipatory process avoiding inappropriate intent. Journal of Advanced Nursing 32(5):1298–1306

Hicks G, Samuels C 2002 Clinical supervision preparation for practice. Gwent Healthcare Training and Development Course Materials, Wales

Jenkins E, Rafferty M, Parke S 2000 Clinical supervision: What is going on in West Wales? Results of a telephone survey. Nursing Times Research 5(1):21–37

Johns C 1993 Professional Supervision. Journal of Nursing Management 1:9–18

Johns C 2002 Guided reflection: advancing practice. Blackwell Science, Oxford, UK

Johns C 2003 Clinical supervision as a model for clinical leadership. Journal of Nursing Management 11(1):25–35

Jones A 1997 A 'bonding between strangers': a palliative model of clinical supervision. Journal of Advanced Nursing 26(5):1028–1035

Jones A 1998 Getting going with clinical supervision: an introductory seminar. Journal of Advanced Nursing 27(3):560–566

Kohner N 1994 Clinical supervision in practice. King's Fund Centre, London

Maggs C 1998 Introducing clinical supervision and beginning evaluation. In: Bishop V (ed) Clinical supervision practice. Macmillan NT Research, Houndmills, Basingstoke, p 40–56

Main T 1989 The hospital as a therapeutic institution (1946). In: Jones J (ed) The ailment and other psychoanalytic essays. Free Association Books, London

Marrow CT, Yaseen et al 1998 Caring together: clinical supervision. Nursing Standard 12 (22 Supplement) 4–18, quiz 20–22

Mattinson S 1975 Reflection process in casework supervision. Tavistock Institute of Marital Studies, London

Nicklin P 1997 A practice-centred model of clinical supervision. Nursing Times 93(46):52–54

NMC 2005 Supporting nurses and midwives through lifelong learning. Nursing Midwifery Council, London, UK

Poulter M, Ball W, Brooks S et al 2005 Clinical supervision/ reflective practice benchmark. East Hampshire NHS Primary Healthcare Trust, Waterlooville, Hampshire, UK

Power S 1999 Nursing supervision: a guide for clinical practice. Sage, London

Proctor B 1986 Supervision: co-operative exercise in accountability. In: Marken M, Payne M (eds) Enabling and ensuring: supervision in practice. National Youth Bureau for Education in Youth and Community Work, Leicester, p 21–23

Proctor B 2001 Training for the supervision alliance attitude, skills and intention. In: Cutcliffe J, Butterworth RT, Proctor B (eds) Fundamental themes in clinical supervision. Routledge, London, p 25–46

Pugsley D, Edwards C 2003 What gets talked about? Clinical supervision: show case programme. Bro Morganwyg NHS Trust (1st November 2003), Wales

Rafferty M 1998 Clinical supervision. In: Barnes E, Griffiths P, Ord J et al (eds) Face to face with distress. Butterworth Heinemann, London

Rafferty M 2000 A conceptual model for clinical supervision in nursing and health visiting based upon Winnicott's (1960) theory of the parent–infant relationship. Journal of Psychiatric and Mental Health Nursing 7(2):153–162

Rafferty M, Jenkins E et al 2003 Developing a provisional standard for clinical supervision in nursing and health visiting: the methodological trail. Qualitative Health Research 13(10):1432–1452

Rafferty M, Jenkins E, Parke S 1998 Clinical supervision: what is going on in West Wales? A report to the clinical effectiveness unit (Wales). The School of Health Science (UWS), Wales

RCN 1999 Realising clinical effectiveness and clinical governance through clinical supervision. An open learning pack. Radclife Medical, Oxford

Rogers C 1962 On becoming a person. Constable, London

Saylor C R 1990 Reflection and professional education: art, science, and competency. Nurse Educator 18(2):8–11

Schon D 1987 The reflective practitioner. Avebury, Aldershot

SCoR 2003 Clinical supervision: a position statement. Society and College of Radiographers, London, UK

Severinsson E, Hallberg I 1996 Clinical supervisors' views of their leadership role in the clinical supervision process within nursing care. Journal of Advanced Nursing 24(1):151–161

Simms J 1993 Supervision. Mental health nursing. Wright and Giddey. Chapman & Hall, London

Sloan G 1998 Clinical supervision: characteristics of a good supervisor. Nursing Standard 12(40):42–46

Snow C, Willard P 1989 I'm dying to take care of you. Professional Counsellor Books, Redmond, WA

Teasdale K, Brocklehurst N, Thom N et al 2001 Clinical supervision and support for nurses: an evaluation study. Journal of Advanced Nursing 33(2):216–224

Thome R 1999 Personal Communication

UKCC 1992 Standards for records and record keeping. UKCC, London

UKCC 1996 Position statement on clinical supervision for nursing and health visiting. United Kingdom Central Council for Nursing, Midwifery and Health Visiting, London, p 1–5

West W 2003 The culture of psychotherapy supervision. Counselling and Psychotherapy Research 3(2):123–127

White E, Winstanley J 2003 Clinical supervision models and best practice. Nurse Researcher 10(4):7–38

Wilkin P, Bowers L, Monk J et al 1997 Clinical supervision: managing the resistance. Nursing Times 93(8):48–49

Winstanley J 2000 Clinical supervision: development of an evaluation instrument. School of Nursing Manchester, University of Manchester

WNB 1994 Discussion document on clinical supervision. Welsh National Board, Cardiff, p 1–6

Wolsey P, Leach L 1997 Clinical supervision: a hornet's nest or honey pot?. Nursing Times 93(44):24–27

Wright S G, Elliott M, Scholefield H et al. (1997) A networking approach to clinical supervision. Nursing Standard 11(18):39–41

Index